MALARIA

A TRAVELLER'S
GUIDE

MALARIA

A TRAVELLER'S GUIDE

originally *A Layman's Guide to Malaria*
by Martine Maurel

COMPLETELY REVISED AND UPDATED BY

DR ANDREW JAMIESON

AND DR STEPHEN TOOVEY

Third edition published by Struik Publishers (a division of New Holland Publishing (South Africa) (Pty) Ltd)
New Holland Publishing is a member of Johnnic Communications Ltd
Cornelis Struik House, 80 McKenzie Street, Cape Town 8001
86 Edgware Road, London, W2 2EA, United Kingdom
14 Aquatic Drive, Frenchs Forest, NSW 2086, Australia
218 Lake Road, Northcote, Auckland, New Zealand
www.struik.co.za

Originally published by Southern Book Publishers in 1994
Second edition published by Struik Publishers in 2001
Copyright © in published edition: Struik Publishers 2001, 2006
Copyright © in text: Martine Maurel 1994

Publishing manager: Linda de Villiers
Editor: Cecilia Barfield
Concept designer: Petal Palmer
Cover designer & DTP: Janine Damon
Proofreader and indexer: Helen de Villiers
Reproduction: Hirt & Carter Cape (Pty) Ltd
Printing and binding: Paarl Print, Oosterland Street, Paarl, South Africa
ISBN 1 77007 353 1
10 9 8 7 6 5 4 3 2 1

www.imagesofafrica.co.za

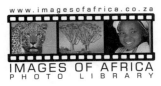

IMAGES OF AFRICA
PHOTO LIBRARY

Log onto our photographic website www.imagesofafrica.co.za for an African experience

DISCLAIMER

Should the reader suspect a malaria condition in himself or any other person, he should make every effort to consult a medical doctor for professional assistance before either treating or not treating himself or that other person. No responsibility will be taken by the author or publisher for any illness or other inconvenience that may result from information given in this book.

DEDICATION

For my beloved son Nicholas who, before his third year of life, grappled five times with the malaria monster and lived to tell the tale.

ACKNOWLEDGEMENTS

I wish to thank Dr Terry Taylor of the Malaria Project Unit at Queen Elizabeth Hospital in Blantyre, Malawi; Dr Eddie Hall, formerly of the Intensive Care Unit at the same hospital; and Dr Gilbert Burnham of Johns Hopkins University, Baltimore, USA, for their invaluable help and encouragement. Grateful thanks also to my commissioning editor, Louise Grantham, for her unwavering faith in the project and to my father, Colin Slater, for his commitment and dedication in guiding the book through to completion.

MARTINE MAUREL
1994

PREFACE

Most doctors in malaria-endemic countries know about malaria. In contrast, doctors in non-malarious countries know very little about it, perhaps understandably. Neither do most ordinary, non-medical people who are likely to come into contact with malaria. This book is for them.

Instead of trying to find out the hard way, through dribs and drabs of information passed on from friend to friend, doctor to patient, and possibly learnt through bitter, frightening experience, your time will be saved if you read this book and keep it as a handy companion on your travels. The knowledge imparted here is readily digestible and not couched in swathes of unintelligible medical jargon.

If you are likely to be placed in a position similar to any of the following scenarios, you will need this book:

- You are the mother of an infant and are visiting a tropical country. Your child has a high fever and you suspect malaria. You are three hours away from a doctor by road and it is midnight. The phone doesn't work or the doctor is not in. What action should you take?

- You are a business traveller and have recently returned to South Africa from a trip to Malawi. Although you took your prophylactics as directed for the duration of your trip and for the recommended period afterwards, it is now four weeks since you have returned home and your bones and joints ache, you have a headache, it is freezing midwinter and your doctor tells you you have a dose of 'flu. You suspect malaria. How can you prove to him that he is wrong?

- You are an expatriate or aid worker living in Kenya, where you are exposed to much expatriate folklore about malaria. You will be living there for three years. Should you take prophylaxis?

- You return to South Africa after a holiday in Zimbabwe. You develop the classic symptoms of malaria but the blood test proves to be negative. Your doctor refuses to treat on the basis of a negative blood test. Time is critical. Should you urge him to treat you anyway?

This book was born out of a baptism of fire. From the age of seven months, my second child suffered five bouts of malaria in one year. The long, lonely hours I spent deep in the night wondering whether he was going to live or die, and knowing that I had conflicting advice from whichever doctor I turned to, prompted me to write this book. Instead of being a mysterious disease to ordinary people who are its victims, malaria needs to be brought out in the open and become understandable.

As the staff of the Malaria Control Unit of the World Health Organization (WHO) point out: 'Ultimately, only people who are well informed (about malaria) hold the key to a malaria-free future.'

Martine Maurel

1994

CONTENTS

INTRODUCTION

Malaria kills three people every minute. Each year, it is thought that as many as 2,7 million people die from malaria and between 300 and 500 million suffer potentially fatal cases. The disease threatens 2,5 billion people, almost half the world's population.

African countries south of the Sahara desert account for 90% of all clinical cases and nearly 90% of deaths caused by malaria. Children are most vulnerable to this major killer. In rural, tropical African areas, one child in 20 dies from malaria before he or she reaches the age of five years.

Despite a ray of hope in the 1960s (when chemical spraying with DDT seemed to control the malaria menace and before it was realized that DDT itself was a killer), reported cases and deaths caused by malaria are rising. For this reason, calls have recently emerged for the limited re-introduction of DDT. Malaria's dramatic resurgence has spurred the WHO to lead two major international initiatives, the Multilateral Initiative on Malaria, and the Roll Back Malaria Initiative.

The Multilateral Initiative on Malaria was announced in Dakar in 1997, and seeks to involve a range of international agencies and organisations in the fight against malaria, while the Roll Back Malaria Initiative, announced in 1998, has set itself dramatic malaria reduction targets.

A number of strategies have been outlined by the WHO to attempt to achieve this control. One of these strategies includes prompt diagnosis and treatment, and this can only be achieved through knowledge and information being made available to the doctor and the patient so that each may recognize malaria in good time.

HOW TO USE THIS BOOK

Note that there is a certain amount of duplication between chapters. Please bear with the author as far as this is concerned as it is intended to simplify the answering of questions for the reader, thus making the book user-friendly. Where pertinent, cross-references to other chapters have been made.

The book is not intended to be read from cover to cover. Rather, it should be used as a reference book: to explain something your doctor mentioned but did not clarify; to answer your urgent questions when a life is at stake and you have no access to medical knowledge; to inform you exactly what the parameters of malaria are, so that it is no longer an awesome, unintelligible disease about which much is speculated.

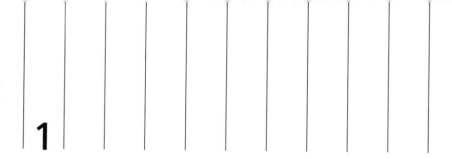

1

WHAT IS MALARIA?

Malaria is a disease, caused by any of four species of parasite, that is carried from person to person by a mosquito and transmitted by the bite of an infected female *Anopheles* mosquito.

Malaria is primarily a disease of the red blood cells and small blood vessels. By causing the cells to become 'sticky' and eventually to burst, it causes blockages of the small blood vessels in the major organs of the body. This can cause severe disease and death – in the case of infection with the *P. falciparum* species of malaria, this can occur within 24 hours of the disease first becoming evident.

Malaria caused by the other three parasites, namely *Plasmodium vivax*, *P. ovale* and *P. malariae,* is much milder and does not cause death, although they cause recurrent malaria that in itself is a debilitating disease.

The malaria parasite is found mostly in the tropical and subtropical regions of the world. Mosquito breeding is severely hampered in temperatures below 20 °C.

Optimal conditions for breeding are at temperatures around 30 °C together with humidity levels of over 60%. Consequently, temperature and humidity largely dictate whether a country is likely to experience year-round malaria, seasonal malaria or localized break throughs.

The severity of malaria and its incidence is governed also by the immunity levels of the host, man. Immunity depends on constant exposure to the malaria-infected mosquito. Hence war and civil disturbances leading to an influx of non-immune workers, as well as tourism, all lead to the exposure of non-immune people to the malaria parasite.

The international consensus of opinion among malaria experts is that non-immune people exposed to malaria should protect themselves against the disease by all possible means. This includes both chemical protection in the form of prophylactics and mechanical protection. Long-term residents of malarious areas, as opposed to short-term travellers, may elect to use personal protection methods alone.

For thousands of years, humans have battled with malaria. Public health has made enormous strides in the management of individual cases of the disease, but the spread of the infection has been aided and abetted by wars, natural disasters, poverty and the emergence of drug and pesticide resistance. Development of candidate vaccines is continuing with limited success; it is unlikely that an effective vaccine will emerge for general usage within the next decade. The most effective means of protection against malaria will remain education, personal protective measures and preventative medication.

The most those of us who are exposed to malaria can do is to arm ourselves with sufficient knowledge of what malaria is all about, to avoid contracting the disease and, if we do contract it, to know how to have it treated promptly and correctly.

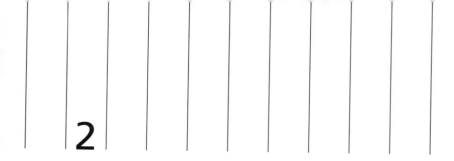

2

THE HISTORY OF MALARIA

Historical records show malaria to be an ancient disease that affected early man as well as certain animals.

In contrast to other diseases with symptoms that have changed over time, the symptoms of malaria have remained the same since they were first recorded more than 2 000 years ago.

MALARIA IN ANCIENT GREECE AND ROME

The ancient Greeks were well acquainted with malaria from about the year 500 BC when infected slaves may have carried the disease into Greece. To a certain extent, malaria may well have contributed to the breakdown of ancient Greek civilisation.

As early as 46 BC, Hippocrates described the malaria symptoms and differentiated between its various forms. However, he incorrectly assumed that malaria was caused as a result of drinking stagnant water.

Some time later, Columella (c. AD 116) linked it with germs breeding in swampy ground and he believed that malaria was transmitted to man by mosquitoes or gnats.

Malaria did not discriminate when choosing its victims. One famous victim was Alexander the Great. Ancient Rome was seen to be vulnerable to the fever to the extent that *Gei Febris*, the fever goddess, was worshipped for her ability to cure the disease. The fall of Rome has been attributed not only to hedonism and decadence, but also to the debilitating effects of the illness on its citizens.

Three emperors, Hadrian, Vespasian and Titus, are believed to have succumbed to malaria, while St Augustine is thought to have contracted it while carrying Christianity's message from Rome to Britain.

Medieval Europe was well acquainted with malaria until land reclamation and improved drainage disrupted the mosquitoes' breeding habits. These habits were further discouraged inadvertently by the increased building of well-lit and ventilated houses.

MALARIA IN ENGLAND

Malaria was commonly known in the English Fens and the marshy Thames Valley. Some of its more famous English victims included James I and Oliver Cromwell. Up until 1859, when the Thames Embankment was built, records show that 5% of admissions to St Thomas' hospital in London were as a result of malaria.

THEORIES ABOUT MALARIA

It took a long time for the connection between malaria and swampy ground to be made. Medieval beliefs that planets and comets rained down a fever-poison or that electrical storms were responsible, had to be overcome first.

During the first half of the nineteenth century it was also believed that dew falling on the decks of ships before sunrise would produce small insects that carried the fever. It was further thought that preferred targets were of fair complexion and were fond of alcohol!

From the Middle Ages up until just over 100 years ago, the dominant theory governing malaria transmission concerned the fact that swamp air contained chemical poisons released from rotting wood. To avoid this, houses were built facing away from wetlands and lakes, and double-storey houses were preferred as it was thought that the air did not rise much above ground level.

Known in the Middle Ages as 'the ague', malaria's connection with marshy ground was entrenched when it was eventually given the Latin name that meant 'bad air', i.e. *mal'aria*.

PROPHYLAXIS

Malaria prophylaxis at the time involved nothing more than the use of crudely made mosquito nets as well as the hanging of garlic and camphor-filled linen bags around the neck.

TREATMENT

Before the discovery of quinine, malaria treatments included lying in steam baths, taking cold dips in the sea, applying blistering equipment, swallowing strychnine, arsenic and large doses of calomel, and the time-honoured application of leeches. Blood-letting was the preferred treatment for fever. Although these were unsuccessful, their use was continued.

THE STORY OF QUININE

Ever since its acceptance in 1640 as a proven remedy for the disease, quinine has been the mainstay of malaria treatment, and still is today. Having observed Peruvians treating malaria successfully, Jesuit priests living in Peru returned to Europe with the bark of a certain tree that, when boiled and the water drunk, greatly improved the survival chances of a malaria victim.

Once introduced to Europe, cinchona (as it was then known) became the drug of choice after use by such famous patients as Charles II and the Archduke Leopold.

Despite its bitter taste and the fact that it sometimes produced deafness, nausea and vomiting, or that its method of action was still mysterious, quinine became known as a miraculous drug.

Its use was linked with serious risks including its association with blackwater fever, an occasional complication of malaria, but known to be one of the commonest causes of death among expatriates in Africa. It is suspected that irregular doses of quinine used as a prophylactic may have caused this much-feared disease.

Today, quinine taken with tetracycline is often the last drug used, after other drugs have failed to quell malaria.

MALARIA IN THE LAST 100 YEARS

DDT was thought to be the great breakthrough of the past 100 years, not for the treatment of malaria, but for its prevention on a mass scale.

Widespread spraying programmes began in the mid-1950s and a marked reduction in the incidence of malaria was experienced in a number of countries. However, it was not until the early 1970s that it was realized to what extent DDT was actually harming the environment.

When it became known that it did not break down into harmless forms but remained harmful for many years, and that, with ingestion, DDT could be passed along the food chain, the distribution of the chemical was banned in many countries and so the incidence of malaria increased. Lately, however, malaria incidence has responded to the limited reintroduction of DDT in certain countries. Used cautiously, it has demonstrated a remarkable ability to reduce the number of malaria cases in high risk areas in local populations. Now that we understand more about the safe use of this pesticide, we can expect that it will be used more widely in the future.

The initial decrease of malaria infections in the late 1960s due to DDT went hand in hand with the introduction of mass prophylaxis campaigns, where populations were treated with chloroquine, as in Tanzania. Here an experiment in mass dosage was carried out where the drug was mixed with table salt in an attempt to ensure that everyone was exposed to it.

Again, it took a while to realize that chloroquine-resistant strains of the parasite were developing as a result of the sub-curative doses used during such mass drug administration. It was still to be realized that mechanical protection was better than chemical protection, at least on a large scale.

Since the mid-1980s, halting the disease's spread seems to have become a lost battle. Between 300 and 500 million people worldwide are affected by malaria each year and it is regarded as a bigger killer than AIDS.

Newer drugs have been under development, including the artemesinin compounds, derived from the Chinese herb *qinghasu*. These compounds, the products of Chinese research, have proved themselves useful in the treatment of malaria when used in combination with older existing drugs. Despite these advances, the hope of eradication has now been transmuted to one merely of control by the WHO.

3

THE WORLDWIDE INCIDENCE OF MALARIA

Worldwide, more than 300 million cases of malaria occur every year – and between 1.5 and 3 million people die as a result. Up to 2.5 billion people in more than 100 countries are exposed to malaria every year. More than 90% of all malaria cases occur in sub-Saharan Africa – remember, though, that malaria also occurs in pockets in tropical and sub-tropical areas in Asia, South and Central America, the Middle East, and Oceania. While these non-African areas make up more than 50% of the area affected by the disease, they are responsible for less than 10% of the cases. But every year, some travellers to these regions and local inhabitants get malaria and a proportion of these die – so the risk should never be underestimated!

Unfortunately, accurate information on the global incidence of malaria is difficult to obtain because reporting of figures, from endemic areas in particular, is incomplete.

At the beginning of the twentieth century, more than two-thirds of the world's population lived in areas where malaria was endemic. Since 1957, concerted efforts at eradication through chemical means have meant that large parts of the globe are now free from malaria.

However, administrative, political and economic obstacles stand in the way of total eradication. Resistance in the mosquito to insecticide and increasing resistance of the malaria parasite to antimalarial drugs add enormously to these obstacles. The widespread resistance of P. falciparum to chloroquine, as reported by national governments around the world to the WHO, has meant that this cheap and generally well-tolerated drug has all but lost its place in our arsenal against the parasite.

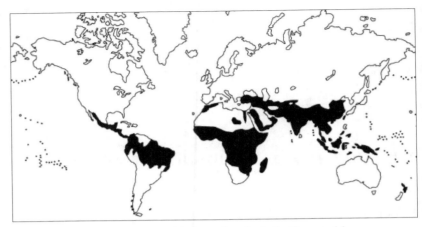

Figure 1: Incidence of malaria in the world

Tables 1A and 1B show countries in which malaria is reported, its incidence, distribution within the country, type of malaria present and resistance (pages 22–29).

Table 1A: African countries, their malaria status and chloroquine resistance (CR) or sensitivity (CS)

Country	Malaria?	CR or CS
Algeria	Yes, but very low risk. No prophylaxis suggested.	
Angola	Yes	CR
Benin	Yes	CR
Botswana	Yes	CR north of Francistown
Burkina Faso	Yes	CR
Burundi	Yes	CR
Cameroon	Yes	CR
Cape Verde	Yes	CR

Central African Republic	Yes	CR
Chad	Yes	CR
Congo	Yes	CR
Djibouti	Yes	CR
Egypt	Yes (limited area – El Faiyum)	CS
Equatorial Guinea	Yes	CR
Eritrea	Whole country <2 000 m	CR – no risk in Asmara
Ethiopia	Whole country <2 000 m	CR, reduced risk in Addis Ababa
Gabon	Yes	CR
Gambia	Yes	CR
Ghana	Yes	CR
Guinea Bissau	Yes	CR
Ivory Coast	Yes	CR
Kenya	Yes	CR
Lesotho	No	
Liberia	Yes	CR
Libya	Very low risk	
Malawi	Yes	CR
Mauritania	Yes	CR
Morocco	Very low risk	
Mozambique	Yes	CR
Namibia	Yes, in north only	CR
Niger	Yes	CR
Nigeria	Yes	CR
Rwanda	Yes	CR
Sao Tomé and Principe	Yes	CR
Senegal	Yes	CR
Sierra Leone	Yes	CR
Somalia	Yes	CR

South Africa	Yes - northen Limpopo, eastern Mpumalanga (whole Kruger Park), and far northen KwaZulu-Natal	
St Helena Is/ Dependencies (incl Ascension, Tristan Da Cunha)	No	
Sudan	Yes	CR
Swaziland	Yes, in Lowveld	CR
Tanzania	Yes	CR
Tunisia	Very low risk	
Uganda	Yes	CR
Zaire	Yes	CR
Zambia	Yes	CR
Zanzibar	Yes	CR
Zimbabwe	Yes	CR, not in Harare or in Highlands

EXPLANATION OF ABBREVIATIONS

CS (Chloroquine Sensitive)   The malaria type is sensitive to chloroquine alone.

CR (Chloroquine Resistant)   The malaria parasite is resistant to chloroquine. Usually Melfloquine or Doxyccline, or Atovaquone plus Proguanil is required. Consult a Travel Clinic for details. Certain medications may not be suitable for all travellers.

Table 1B: Other countries in which malaria is a threat to health, its incidence, distribution within the country, principal species present, and resistance

Country	Time	Altitude	Location	P. vivax	P. falciparum	Resistant to
ASIA						
Azerbaijan	Jun–Sep		Rural lowland areas	Exclusive		
Bangladesh	All year		Entire country except Dhaka		Predominant	Chloroquine S/P
Cambodia	All year		Entire country except Phnom Penh & Tonle Sap		Predominant	Chloroquine S/P Mefloquine on border
China	Jul–Nov north of 33 °N May–Dec 25 °N–33 °N All year south of 25 °N only	<1 500 m	In general, in remote rural areas in the south west	Focal	Predominant	Multidrug resistance has been reported

Country	Time	Altitude	Location	P. vivax	P. falciparum	Resistant to
India	All year	<2 000 m	Most of country including cities			
Indonesia	All year		Entire country excl Jakarta, big cities, & tourist resorts in Bali & Java	Resistant P. vivax in Irian Java	Predominant	Chloroquine S/P
Laos	All year		Entire country except Vientiane		Predominant	Chloroquine
Malaysia	All year		Limited foci in deep hinterland & Sabah		Predominant	Chloroquine S/P
Myanmar (Burma)	All year	<1 000 m	Karen State		Predominant	Chloroquine S/P
	Seasonal		Other areas		Predominant	Chloroquine S/P
Nepal	All year		Rural low-lying areas <2 000 m	Present	Present	Chloroquine
Tajikistan	Jun–Oct			Predominant	Present	Chloroquine

Country	Time	Altitude	Location	P. vivax	P. falciparum	Resistant to
Thailand	All year		Rural, forested, hilly areas only – not tourist areas	Present	Predominant	Chloroquine S/P Mefloquine on borders
Vietnam	All year		Entire country except urban areas, Red River Delta, Nha Trang		Predominant	Chloroquine S/P
SOUTH AMERICA						
Argentina	Oct–May mainly	<1 200 m	Rural borders with Bolivia & Paraguay	Exclusive		
Belize	All year		Entire country	91%	9%	
Brazil	All year	<900 m	Especially mining & agricultural areas in Amazon region	77%	23%	Chloroquine S/P
Colombia	All year	<800 m	Rural areas	54%	46%	Chloroquine S/P
Dominican Republic	All year		Rural areas in west		Predominant	

Country	Time	Altitude	Location	P. vivax	P. falciparum	Resistant to
Ecuador	All year	<1 500 m	Entire country except Quito & Guayaquil	49%	51%	Chloroquine
French Guiana	All year		Entire country, but mainly in south		Predominant	Multidrug resistant
Nicaragua	All year		Most of country	Pre-dominant		
Surinam	All year		Entire country, mainly in south		Predominant	Chloroquine S/P
Venezuela	All year		Rural areas	Present	Jungle areas mainly	Chloroquine

MIDDLE EAST

Country	Time	Altitude	Location	P. vivax	P. falciparum	Resistant to
Iraq	May– Nov	<1 500 m	In the north	Exclusive		
Oman	All year		Remote areas only		Predominant	Chloroquine

Country	Time	Altitude	Location	P. vivax	P. falciparum	Resistant to
Syria	May – Oct		North only	Exclusive		
Turkey	May – Oct		Mainly south-east	Predominant		
ISLANDS						
Papua New Guinea	All year	<1 800 m	Entire country		Predominant	Chloroquine S/P
Solomon Islands	All year		Nearly entire country		Predominant	Chloroquine S/P
Vanuatu	All year		Entire country		Predominant	Chloroquine S/P

4

THE MOSQUITO

More than 3 200 species of mosquito have been identified. Not all carry malaria, but of those that do, some species transmit it to humans more efficiently than others. Only the genus *Anopheles* carries a malaria parasite that can be transmitted to human beings.

FEEDING AND BREEDING HABITS

Female adult mosquitoes feed on human and animal blood, the male mosquito feeds on plant nectar. In order to breed, one needs plants for the male mosquito to thrive – therefore reducing flowering plants reduces the mosquito population. Water is required, sometimes in surprisingly small quantities, for the eggs to hatch and larvae to develop – so, reducing freestanding water makes a big difference in keeping mosquitoes away from your residence.

Mosquitoes always breed in water or damp locations. Eggs are deposited on damp soil or vegetation, in moist tree holes and containers or sometimes directly onto water, from where the larvae hatch.

Optimal breeding temperatures for mosquitoes are between 25 °C and 30 °C. They can still breed in temperatures as low as 20 °C but cooler conditions will severely hamper the hatching of larvae. Ideal conditions are in humidity levels greater than 60%.

The majority of mosquitoes hunt and feed at night. Each species has a well-defined activity cycle with some attacking at dusk and others at around midnight.

WHEN DO THEY NORMALLY BITE?

The *Anopheles* females, which carry malaria, require a blood-meal in order to feed their developing eggs. They are night feeders – so you are at risk from dusk to dawn. Some areas have mosquitoes that bite at differing times at night – for example, African mosquitoes often bite most between 22h00 and 04h00; the importance of mosquito nets in this environment becomes obvious. But remember you can be bitten at any time at night, and there are even reports of *Anopheles* mosquitoes biting in heavily shaded and dark areas in the day.

WHAT KIND OF ACTIVITY CYCLES DO THEY DISPLAY?

Some mosquitoes feed only outdoors, but the majority feed indoors. After feeding, they like to sit on the walls and ceilings – so it stands to reason that spraying walls and ceilings with long-lasting insecticide will be of benefit. In fact – this is the basis of many mosquito control programmes – its called 'indoor residual insecticide spraying'. Similarly spraying under and behind furniture helps to kill mosquitoes in their daytime resting areas.

THEIR MOVEMENTS AND THE LINK WITH RESISTANCE

Mosquitoes are accomplished flyers and are able to disperse over an area of a few kilometres. However, most species remain in rather restricted habitats, usually near to their larval development site. This would explain why even when resistance in a person is built up, that resistance is usually only to the type of parasite carried by the mosquitoes living in a particular area. That same person is not likely to be resistant to malaria in a different region.

REDUCING YOUR CHANCES OF BEING BITTEN BY CHANGING YOUR ENVIRONMENT

It has been suggested that the likelihood of getting bitten by a malaria-carrying mosquito may be reduced if you ensure that you do not choose holiday accommodation in an area near a large number of children as they usually carry a high proportion of malaria parasites in their bodies when they are infected; neither should you have maize, sisal or bananas or any other dense vegetation growing in your garden or near your house, as these may act as resting sites for mosquitoes. Small amounts of water can be enough for mosquitoes to breed – an upturned leaf, long grass, a footprint or a bottle top can hold enough water. Strict tidiness and hygiene around the home really does pay off in malaria control.

WHAT DOES THE *ANOPHELES* MOSQUITO LOOK LIKE?

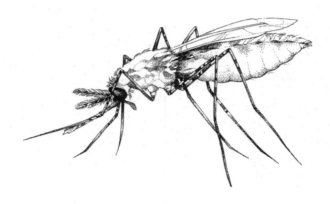

HOW DOES IT LOCATE ITS PREY?

Anopheles is blind in the dark but seeks its host in response to a combination of chemical and physical stimuli. It has sensors in its two antennae that enable it to detect the stream of carbon dioxide exhaled by its prey, and it detects chemicals given off by people when they sweat. Pregnant women, for instance, give off chemicals that make them very attractive to mosquitoes – increasing their risk of malaria.

This allows it to calculate its distance from the prey as it moves towards it through the changing concentrations in the air of warmth, moisture and the ingredients of human sweat.

Human perspiration differs in its content, with that of certain individuals being more desirable to the biting insect than that of others. This may explain to a limited extent why certain people are bitten more often than others.

DOES THE MALARIA-CARRYING MOSQUITO MAKE A NOISE?

In contrast to the relatively high-pitched, loud, characteristic whine of the mosquito, the malaria-carrying mosquito has a low-pitched, almost inaudible hum, unless it is quite close to the ear.

WHAT CAUSES THE ITCHY BITE?

A localized sensitivity to saliva from the mosquito causes the itch. The saliva contains an anti-clotting agent that allows the blood-meal to enter the mosquito's stomach without coagulating and becoming indigestible.

The same reaction seems to be present with all types of mosquito but the size of the reaction seems to differ in varying degrees, i.e. some bites may be visible for days, while others disappear about half an hour after the person has been bitten; some cause a lot of itching while others hardly at all.

HOW DOES IT FEED?

Highly adapted to its job of sucking blood efficiently, the mosquito has a proboscis or long, sucking organ, consisting of six hair-like stylets or probes, two of which are used for piercing the skin, while two saw the wound open and the third pair suck out the blood-feed. This occurs only after a minute amount of saliva has been injected through them into the wound. Some people have made the mistake of thinking they haven't been bitten – no itchy bite, no mosquitoes heard – and have stopped their medication, only to develop malaria.

5

THE DIFFERENT TYPES OF MALARIA

The four types of malaria are split into two categories; there are three types that are benign forms: *Plasmodium vivax*, *P. malariae* and *P. ovale*, and one malignant form: *Plasmodium falciparum*. The latter parasite is responsible for the majority of deaths caused by malaria, whereas the malaria caused by the first three do not usually cause death, but only debilitating disease, which in some cases can recur over many years.

One reason for the difference in severity can be attributed to the various parasites' preference for red blood cells at different stages of maturation: while *P. malariae* prefers mature blood cells, *P. vivax* and *P. ovale* invade younger red blood cellss; *P. falciparum*, on the other hand, is indiscriminate in its choice of red blood cells, hence its form of attack is all-encompassing. This substantially broadens the scope and potential severity of its attack.

Another reason why *P. falciparum* is so deadly, is that for each liver cell invaded by a single malaria parasite after the mosquito bite, around 40 000 parasites are released 10 to14 days later. This compares to far fewer – 2 000 to 5 000 – in the forms of malaria.

The life cycles of the four malarial parasite types are broadly similar, with different stages of development occurring in appropriate female *Anopheles* mosquito hosts as well as in the human host.

The least dangerous form of the disease causes periodic chills and fevers but is rarely fatal, hence the term 'benign'. Despite the term 'benign', *P. vivax* malaria can be fatal in patients who suffer traumatic rupture of the spleen and in those who develop severe anaemia, especially malnourished and debilitated patients.

Old-fashioned terms for the different types of malaria are:

P. vivax	Benign tertian, simple tertian, tertian
P. malariae	Quartan
P. falciparum	Malignant tertian, subtertian, aestivo-autumnal, tropical pernicious
P. ovale	Ovale tertian

These colloquial names have become largely obsolete.

PLASMODIUM VIVAX

After *P. falciparum, P. vivax* is the second most widely experienced form of malaria. A serious complication in untreated infections is rupture of the spleen as noted above. *P. Vivax* occurs mostly in the temperate zone as well as in the tropics. It is common in Central America and China where it is responsible for most malaria cases, whereas in West Africa and East Africa it causes only about 2% of malaria cases.

To demonstrate how benign it is, of the more than five million cases of *vivax* malaria epidemic in Sri Lanka in 1969, not one person died. Moreover, this type of malaria is associated with people of a certain blood type not usually found in Africans.

Characteristically, it causes malaria with frequent relapses if not treated properly, the pattern of which varies in relation to the various strains of *P. vivax*. The incubation period between the time of the first infected bite to first onset of symptoms is between 12 and 17 days or even up to a year, depending on the strain involved. The severity of the first attack ranges from mild to severe depending on the immune responses of the host and the degree of parasite infection, i.e. for victims with no immunity, severity is likely to be marked.

PLASMODIUM OVALE

This type of malaria is more commonly encountered in sub-Saharan Africa than the *P. vivax* type. It has mostly been found in West Africa.

Its symptoms are indistinguishable from those of *P. vivax* and *P. malariae*, the other benign types of malaria.

Characteristically, it produces fever spikes every 48 to 50 hours but this may differ markedly with different cases. If left untreated, or treated inadequately, the infection typically lasts from 18 months to three years although periods of recurrence may be lengthy between attacks.

The severity of the first attack is typically mild with fever attacks lasting from eight to 12 hours.

Incubation from the time of the first infected bite until onset of symptoms is typically from 16 to 18 days or even longer (depending on the strain involved).

PLASMODIUM MALARIAE

Also known as *malariae quartain* as its fevers sometimes spike every 72 hours. Its course is not unduly severe but it is notorious for its long persistence in the body if adequate treatment is not given. Its geographical range extends over both tropical and subtropical areas.

The incubation period between the time of the first infected bite and the first onset of symptoms ranges between 18 and 40 days or even longer.

This can present problems in those who, for instance, get bitten on the last day of their holiday and develop malaria symptoms some five weeks later. Unless one was looking out for malaria, it would be difficult to immediately link the illness with the holiday. This is compounded because the severity of the first attack is usually so mild that it may arouse little suspicion.

The fever cycle usually occurs every 72 hours while the fever lasts for an average of eight to ten hours.

P. malariae does not relapse as happens with *P. vivax* and *P. ovale*, but rather 'recrudesces' or 'breaks through' again. With the *P. malariae* parasite it seems that the infection persists in very low concentrations in the blood. When the concentration increases we say that the infection has 'recrudesced'. The incidence of break throughs is high and these can last for between three and 50 years.

It is possible for the host to be infected and not develop symptoms for 50 years, as happened in one case where a person who had lived in a malarious area briefly in his youth developed it many years later after spending the rest of his life in non-malarious England. The reason for such a long, symptom-free period is unknown, nor has it been confirmed that stress or illness may have a part to play in triggering the disease.

PLASMODIUM FALCIPARUM

Malignant malaria, the killer disease, is caused by the species named *Plasmodium falciparum*, which nearly always causes severe, life-threatening malaria in non-immune hosts. The greater the amount of immunity possessed by the host, the milder the disease is when it does strike. Over 90% of malaria cases and 90% of deaths in Africa are due to *P. falciparum* whereas about 40% of total cases in Asia are due to it.

P. falciparum malaria is the fatal form of malaria that can kill a non-immune person within less than a week or two of a primary attack, unless appropriate treatment is given in time. It takes between six and 21 days for malaria to develop from the time of the first infected bite to the first sign or symptom. In this time the parasite has been multiplying in the liver before being released into the bloodstream and invading the red blood cells.

The typical cycle between fever spikes is usually 48 hours, but with different batches of parasite maturing at different times, these fever spikes are likely to become less obvious and interspersed with other fever spikes, making detection of a pattern difficult.

The severity of *P. falciparum* malaria in those adults and children who have it for the first time is severe and may be fatal. Children who survive repeated attacks of malaria in an area do develop a measure of resistance (called semi-immunity) that persists into adulthood. If the region is left, though, the resistance rapidly wanes. As a rule, adults do not usually develop semi-immunity.

Should a relapse occur as a result of inadequate or incorrect treatment of the malaria attack, it will break out again relatively soon, i.e. a few weeks. While *P. falciparum* is by far the most dangerous form of malaria, a feature of this strain is that if adequately treated, it should not recur – unlike *P. vivax* and *P. ovale*.

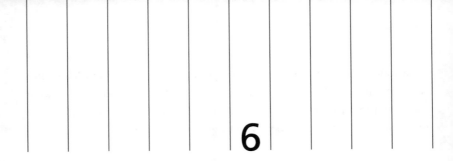

THE SYMPTOMS OF MALARIA

The symptoms of malaria are the same today as they were more than 2 000 years ago when they were first described. The static nature of these symptoms contrasts with other diseases whose symptoms have varied over time.

GENERAL SYMPTOMS

The symptoms are basically similar for all four types of malaria, although the clinical manifestations may differ significantly. In general, the infection is characterized by bouts of fever occurring at regular intervals, alternating with periods of partial recovery with the patient becoming weaker as time goes on.

It is important to note that the classic description is characteristic but *not* universal, and that variations may be found, which typically serve to confuse diagnosis.

When malaria strikes, the most characteristic feature is that of an intermittent fever. Although a pattern of recurring fever may be discernible, it should not be relied on by patient or clinician to help with the diagnosis.

As the fever rises, attacks of rigors occur. These involve a feeling of bone-chilling cold that may seem absolutely ridiculous to the observer – the room temperature may be 35° C and everyone else feels uncomfortably hot, while the malaria sufferer simply cannot warm up!

After peaking – either naturally, or after the administration of medication to alleviate the fever – the patient's temperature will begin to drop, and at that stage he or she will fling off all blankets and coverings, and feel unbearably hot.

This is usually followed by a period of sweating, which can be quite spectacular. Although the malaria sufferer feels better in this phase, often falling asleep, large volumes of fluid can be lost as clothes and bedding are saturated. As the liver and spleen become enlarged, abdominal pain may occur. Vomiting and diarrhoea may occur, and add to dehydration and low blood pressure. Headache is almost always present, and patients complain of very severe tiredness and lassitude.

Children often present differently to adults. Paroxysms of fever are not as common as with adults, while headache, nausea, vomiting, abdominal pain, diarrhoea, a sustained fever and convulsions make up a much less characteristic clinical picture.

WHAT MAKES DIAGNOSIS DIFFICULT?

Diagnosis is particularly difficult with children who may have high blood levels of parasite infection but relatively mild symptoms.

Conversely, there may be little or no sign of parasites in the blood and symptoms may be severe.

Misdiagnosis is a serious problem in areas where health workers are not familiar with malaria, or with patients in whom the range of symptoms may not clearly point to malaria.

SYMPTOMS OF *PLASMODIUM FALCIPARUM*

The incubation period of *P. falciparum* malaria is usually between seven and 12 days and is seldom over 28 days (although cases of longer duration have been recorded).

The onset of malaria may be quite distinctive and unmistakable in some persons, while in others it may be slow and non-specific, causing medical care not to be sought for several days. However, the first attack of *P. falciparum* in non-immune patients is the most serious and dangerous, because the host has no immunity against the disease and is at his or her most vulnerable. These patients may have a 'flu-like' illness, with fever, headache, dizziness, malaise, aches and pains, although shaking chills and high fever are not always present.

Jaundice, which is not uncommon, may be mistaken for viral hepatitis. Associated symptoms vary, but may also include nausea, vomiting and a bronchitic cough. Diarrhoea is not uncommon.

The character of the fever, its symptoms and course are irregular and variable. At first, the fever is intermittent and irregular; later it is characterized by numerous peaks representing the activity of different groups of parasites.

Anaemia arises from the destruction of the red blood cells by the malaria parasite. The *P. falciparum* parasite shows no discrimination in blood cells and will destroy cells of any age, as opposed to the *P. vivax* parasite, which destroys only young or immature blood cells. Each red blood cell invaded releases 20 to 32 new parasites when it bursts – a simple calculation will show how rapidly the parasites can multiply; in three generations one parasite will give rise to around 32 000 new ones. This is why *P. falciparum* malaria can bring a person to death's door within hours.

This blanket approach explains why the patient will deteriorate far more quickly than he would with the other forms of malaria. The invasion of the red blood cells causes them to stick together forming small clots that block capillaries, leading to areas of defective oxygenation in many tissues. It is also thought that a toxic substance is produced by *P. falciparum* that may possibly adversely affect the metabolism of the tissue cells.

Taken together, the results of *P. falciparum* infection can be sudden, grave and can develop without warning. These complications include cerebral malaria (see section on Complications, pages 64–68).

THE RECURRING MALARIAS

P. vivax and *P. ovale* types of malaria recur because the parasite incubates in the liver for long periods after infection and then appears in the blood, causing renewed symptoms on relapse. This may explain why the patient can undergo attacks long after he has left the malarious area.

SYMPTOMS OF *PLASMODIUM VIVAX*

The variable incubation lasts between nine and 15 days after which a classic three-stage attack cycle begins. *P. vivax* is characterized by a primary attack followed by relapses until the patient is cured. It is a serious illness that can lead to anaemia and debility but it is not life threatening.

The spleen usually enlarges rapidly in *P. vivax malaria*, and may after repeated infections be massively enlarged. The few people who do die of vivax malaria usually do so after minor abdominal injuries, causing the spleen to burst with subsequent internal bleeding.

Anaemia results from the destruction of the red blood cells and this may be severe in children. In severe cases, jaundice may develop. Anaemia may become a significant problem in pregnancy, and placental problems may occur, leading to premature labour or miscarriage.

Relapses usually fall into two categories: early (eight to 10 weeks after the attack) and late (between 30 and 40 weeks after the attack).

SYMPTOMS OF *PLASMODIUM MALARIAE* (QUARTAN)

Incubation is between 15 and 40 days and is followed by a three-stage cycle of similar severity to that in *P. vivax* infection but which occurs at 72-hour intervals. Patients have been known to experience relapses up to 20 years after the primary infection.

This infection can be completely wiped out by adequate retreatment so that relapses do not occur. It is not life threatening although it can cause kidney complications.

SYMPTOMS OF *PLASMODIUM OVALE* (TERTIAN)

This is much milder than a *P. vivax* infection, and it exhibits similar symptoms. In the primary attack, the fever occurs at 48-hour intervals.

7

THE LIFE CYCLE OF THE MALARIA PARASITE

After a mosquito carrying malaria parasites has bitten a person, the parasites have been shown to disappear from the outer (peripheral) blood supply within half an hour, only to return to it six to 16 days later. During this week-long latent period, the malarial patient cannot re-infect a 'clean' mosquito if he or she is bitten again.

Soon after entering the human bloodstream, the parasites 'hide' in the host's liver, where they are largely immune to drug therapy. For the next period, until they emerge from the liver – between six days and as long as two years – they are only treatable by drugs that can attack the liver stage. These drugs are called 'Causal prophylactics or treatments', and include atovaquone/proguanil and primaquine.

After lodging in the liver for six to 15 days, the parasites multiply and are released into the bloodstream. There they invade red blood cells where they multiply and are released into the bloodstream, where the process continues. As it continues, the infection leads to a progressive increase of parasites into the blood (parasitaemia) until the process is slowed down by the immune response of the host, is blocked by appropriate treatment, or ultimately overwhelms the system and results in death.

This development takes 48 hours in tertian malaria (i.e. in three different types of parasite – P. falciparum, P. vivax and P. ovale) to 72 hours in quartan malaria (P. malariae).

P. vivax, P. malariae and P. ovale are very specific in terms of the red blood cells they attack. This is one of the reasons why they result in correspondingly less severe pathological changes and manifestations than

The mosquito bites its victim.

Malaria parasite sporozoites in the salivary gland are injected into the person's bloodstream.

The parasite heads for the liver cells where it stays for an incubatory phase for between six and 15 days. *P. ovale* and *P. vivax* stay dormant in the liver for much longer.

In the liver, parasites develop into another form (schizonts) which, in turn, mature and release a differentiated form of parasite (merozoite) into the bloodstream where they invade red blood cells. At this point, in *P vivax* and *ovale*, some of these meroziotes reinvade the liver and go into hiding, causing future relapses.

Some of the newly released merozoites are differentiated into gametocytes.

In the bloodstream (the bloodstream form) they mature into schizonts and are released as merozoites from the red blood cell when it ruptures. This causes fever.

These, while circulating in the bloodstream, are ingested when a mosquito takes a blood-feed from the person.

The released merozoites invade new blood cells, causing the fever. The process continues until death or appropriate medication kills the parasite.

A further form of parasite development and differentiation takes place inside the mosquito resulting in the beginning of the cycle again when the parasite lodges in the salivary glands of the mosquito and gets injected into humans when they are bitten again.

N.B. Different drugs are effective at different stages in the parasite's life cycle.

Figure 2: The life cycle of the malaria parasite

happens with *P. falciparum*. The latter invades any red blood cells resulting in severe and sudden symptoms in some individuals. Infections of *P. vivax* and *P. ovale* malarias may remain in a dormant phase on entering the liver and only begin active division after a genetically predetermined interval, causing the characteristic relapses of these infections.

As parasites continue to multiply, the red blood cells become sticky and clump together. This causes small blood vessels to become blocked, affecting the brain, lungs and kidneys. When they eventually rupture, they release various substances into the blood that cause pain and fever.

When a certain number of blood cells are destroyed, anaemia with jaundice may develop.

Characteristically, the spleen and liver may become enlarged as a result of increased debris from the digested and ruptured red blood cells.

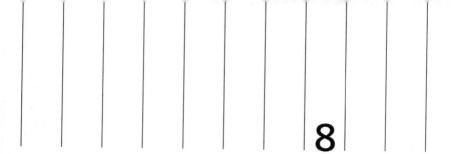

8

WHAT TO DO IF MALARIA IS SUSPECTED

Malaria is unique in its propensity to pass rapidly from a mild illness whose treatment is relatively simple, to a catastrophic state in which the outlook is virtually hopeless.

Failure to consider malaria in diagnosis, or the inability to recognize parasites in a blood smear, can prove fatal.

SYMPTOMS

The signs that should alert you to a possibility of malaria include those that are described under the sections on symptoms (pages 38–41).

However, remember that in some cases, fever may not be present, while only diarrhoea and/or vomiting may be present. If you feel unwell, especially 'fluey', and you have recently been or are living in a country where malaria is endemic, you should first of all consider the possibility of malaria.

TESTING

Rather test for it and come up with negative results than assume that something else is wrong with you. However, to complicate matters, also remember that if you are taking prophylactics, your test may well initially come up negative.

TIME IS OF THE ESSENCE

Remember, time is of the essence. If malaria is suspected early in the evening, and it is decided that a doctor will be consulted only the next morning, a whole 12 hours will have elapsed during which time the parasite can multiply and significantly weaken someone who is at risk, i.e. a baby or a small child, a pregnant woman, or a non-immune person.

WHAT IF YOU CANNOT GET HOLD OF A DOCTOR?

It is best to consult whatever medical facilities are likely to be open at the time or to take the decision to treat for malaria yourself. Having a malaria rapid test kit on hand enables you to test yourself for malaria. These tests are not universally accurate, and users may make mistakes – but they do help in those instances where people feel mildly unwell and are uncertain what to do. A negative test should never stop you from taking treatment if you are unable to consult a doctor and your symptoms are consistent with malaria. Remember that other serious infections, such as typhoid, may occur in malaria endemic areas – not every fever is malaria. Once you decide to treat for malaria, you need to have on hand one of the treatment drugs recommended for that particular region.

It is essential that you seek medical advice as soon as possible to confirm the diagnosis and to confirm that you are taking the correct drug regimen. If medical help is not available, your best course would be to take the entire course of treatment as prescribed in the package insert of the drug.

If your condition worsens then you can assume one of two things: you are suffering from malaria but the drug you have taken has not worked and you have to take a more powerful drug. Or, you are not suffering from malaria at all, but rather from some other disease on which the drugs you have taken have no effect.

WHAT DRUGS SHOULD YOU HAVE ON HAND?

Quinine, followed by a second drug such as doxycycline, will prove a reliable and effective cure in most situations. For uncomplicated cases of malaria, co-artemether (artemether and benflumetol) will provide a rapid relief of symptoms and a reliable cure. Despite being commonly offered alone in Africa and Asia, artemether should always be used in combination. The existence of widespread resistance to chloroquine and sulphadoxine/ pyrimethamine effectively rules out chloroquine as a first-line choice of treatment. Refer to pages 62–63 for the first-line drug of choice for treatment.

Fever is likely to persist for as long as 48 to 72 hours with most forms of treatment before improvement is noted. With co-artemether, fever may subside a lot quicker, but the full course of treatment should nevertheless be completed.

Between the time the dose was given and the next morning there may still be some effect of a failed or inadequate drug, enough to hold off multiplication of the parasite until a doctor is consulted.

The doctor must advise you whether to continue with the drug, how to watch out for signs that the drug was not working and when to come back for a further blood test to ascertain that the parasite had been eradicated from the bloodstream. Repeat blood tests after 24 to 36 hours are important.

OTHER MEASURES TO HELP MINIMIZE THE EFFECTS OF MALARIA
Other measures that should be taken include giving antifever drugs, such as paracetamol. Avoid aspirin and anti-inflammatories as this may interfere with blood flow through the kidneys. Have sugar-containing drinks and sweets on hand, as blood sugar may drop in malaria – this is worse when quinine is taken. Additionally, taking one or two doses of antinausea agents such as cyclizine may help with vomiting.

If the patient is vomiting, note when the drug was given and whether enough time elapsed (one hour) before the vomiting started. If vomiting has occurred within 45 minutes of taking the medication, it should be repeated.

DRUG ADMINISTRATION AND ABSORPTION
Medical opinion is divided on the specific time that should be allowed to elapse after the medicine has been taken, and before vomiting occurs, to

judge if absorption has taken place. Absorption depends on whether food was present in the stomach at the time of ingestion or not; on the metabolic rate of the particular patient; and on the drug that is administered.

If insufficient time for absorption occurred, then the dose must be re-administered. Overdosage has different effects with different drugs. If vomiting is already established or if the patient is prone to vomiting, give the patient an anti-nausea, anti-vomiting drug about 45 minutes before you are due to give the medication.

Unfortunately very few treatment drugs are available in suppository form at present – something that would go a long way to overcoming the problem of vomiting and having to put the patient on a drip.

Remember that if diarrhoea is present as well, the patient must be rehydrated adequately.

Table 2: Rehydration therapy

Large amounts of fluid or oral rehydrate solution (ORS) are to be taken in cases of diarrhoea to ensure adequate rehydration (recommended by the WHO)

Children less than two years:
    50 ml to 100 ml after each loose stool
Children two to 10 years:
    100 ml to 200 ml after each loose stool
Older children to adults:
    Unlimited amounts

If ORS is not available, make up a home-made solution:
    Six level tablespoons of sugar
    One level teaspoon of salt
    Dissolve the above in one litre of clean, boiled water.
Drink this in amounts as indicated above for ORS.

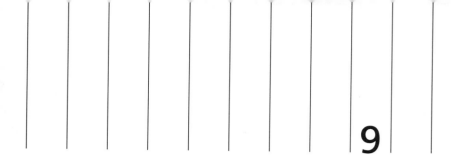

9

DIAGNOSIS

Most deaths in short-stay travellers, which are due to malaria, are likely to occur after their return to their country of origin. The single biggest contributory factor in the death of such a person is *the lack of prompt and accurate diagnosis*.

Indeed, in 1993 the family of a man who died of malaria in an English hospital after returning from Kenya, successfully sued the hospital for failure to diagnose malaria. The award granted was £900 000.

Doctors in non-endemic areas may not be alert to a diagnosis of malaria, nor be familiar with the disease. Even if blood smears are taken for some other reason, malarial parasites may not be recognized by lab technicians as they will not be looking for them, nor will they have any experience in recognizing them.

It is also necessary to guard against the possibility of your blood test being sent away to another hospital for analysis. Inquire how long it will be before you have the results. One hapless person returning to the United Kingdom, who suspected he might have malaria, had the foresight to have his blood tested. Unfortunately, he received his results three days later, during which time he may easily have died had his results been positive.

This applies in particular to school children who return to school in England or some other European country after spending a holiday with their parents in a malaria-endemic area. School masters and school doctors need to be very alert in their diagnosis of fevers in such children on their return to school.

One wise rule is to make sure the traveller returning from a malaria zone is equipped with an effective treatment drug in case they meet with any difficulty or delay in obtaining the drug in their home country.

Be on your guard if you or your visitors leave the malaria zone and, within a month to six weeks, come down with what seems like 'flu. It is so easy to forget that you have been in an endemic area and that malaria may be the cause of your illness.

BASING DIAGNOSIS ON A BLOOD SMEAR

If there is suspicion on the doctor's part that malaria may be present, he should begin antimalarial therapy *even if parasites are not found in the blood smear*. It has been known for doctors who are not familiar with malaria to refuse to treat for malaria despite all the classic symptoms being present, unless they can see parasites in the blood smear.

It may be that the parasites at an early stage of development in the body may not be visible in the peripheral bloodstream, making a blood smear inconclusive. If this is the case, examinations of blood smears taken at frequent intervals may be necessary to establish a diagnosis.

It is not easy to say exactly, but two or three blood smears taken every eight to 12 hours should be sufficient to confirm diagnosis.

To complicate the issue, a positive blood smear taken from a feverish patient living in an endemic region does not conclusively implicate malaria as the cause of the illness. This is because the patient may show no symptoms but may have parasites circulating in the blood anyway. His immunity may be such that the infection is under control and not causing disease. In such a case the patient's fever may be due to other infectious agents.

Research has repeatedly shown that malaria is over-diagnosed in Africa. This is due to a number of factors, such as fear of leaving undiagnosed malaria untreated, substandard equipment and stains, and overwork, to name a few. If a 'malaria' does not show signs of settling, then be prepared to consider another diagnosis. In addition, patients with cerebral malaria may display scanty parasite counts while many children with high parasite counts may display fairly mild symptoms.

Patients who have been taking prophylactics need to tell their doctors this, as these may well mask the presence of parasites in the blood and result in a seemingly negative blood smear. The conclusion therefore is that a negative blood smear does not exclude malaria and a positive blood smear does not necessarily confirm a diagnosis of malaria.

A good rule of thumb to apply is the following: malaria should be suspected by medical personnel in anyone with a fever who has recently been in a malaria-endemic area. The doctor should admit the patient to hospital for drug administration by drip if the patient is unable to keep down medication given by mouth.

Admission to the intensive care unit should be made if the patient:
- has difficulty in talking
- has difficulty sitting up
- has difficulty standing
- has difficulty walking without any obvious cause e.g. unexplained heavy bleeding, the passing of small quantities of, or no, urine, or the passage of dark urine
- displays a change of behaviour
- seems confused
- seems drowsy
- displays altered consciousness or coma
- is suffering from jaundice and/or severe anaemia
- is suffering from circulatory collapse or shock
- has difficulty in breathing

Severe *P. falciparum* malaria is a medical emergency demanding the highest level of care and treatment available in an intensive care unit.

WHAT SHOULD YOU TELL YOUR DOCTOR?

You should tell him or her whether you have been travelling in or visiting a malarial area and when you were there. Your doctor also needs to know whether you have had any symptoms in the past that may have been attributable to malaria and whether you have any history of liver disorder, as this may complicate matters tremendously.

Inform your doctor if you are/may be pregnant and whether you are breastfeeding. Tell him or her which prophylactic drugs, if any, you had been taking for malaria and for how long, whether you took the whole dosage conscientiously, and whether you have attempted any self treatment.

If your doctor is unfamiliar with malaria, ask him or her to make contact with a centre of excellence regarding malaria in the country you are in, for further advice.

GUIDELINES FOR THE MANAGEMENT OF MALARIA

The following details the sequence of events that may be used by a clinician in the management of malaria; nuances may vary but the basic principles are similar. The purpose of this section is to give you insight into the thought processes of your doctor, not to equip you to treat malaria yourself.

The essence of successful malaria case management is early treatment. To achieve this requires awareness of the symptoms and the importance of being tested without delay.

Possible malaria

Any person who feels unwell in a malaria area should be tested for malaria – any or all of the following symptoms must be regarded as malaria until proven otherwise:

- Headache
- Muscle aches
- Joint pain
- Nausea
- Vomiting
- Diarrhoea
- Cough
- Sore throat
- Tiredness/fatigue
- Hot and cold shivers
- Fever

TESTING FOR MALARIA

- No symptoms or physical signs are specific for malaria i.e. they can be present in any number of ways that mimic common flu to more serious illness.
- The only certain way to diagnose malaria is to perform tests that are specific for malaria.
- There are basically two tests available in most malarious areas .

Rapid tests

- These are sensitive and reliable enough to be used by anybody with minimal basic training.
- No specialised equipment or laboratory facilities are required.
- They are also portable and temperature stable enough to be transported and stored at indoor room temperature without special facilities.
- Combination type tests are best as they differentiate between potentially fatal *P. falciparum* and the three less dangerous other types of malaria.
- The test procedure must be according to the manufacturer's instructions.

Blood slides (done in laboratory)

Blood smears are the gold standard of malaria tests, because:

- False negative results are uncommon in good hands.
- The species of malaria can be identified.
- The parasite count can be determined, which is important in decision making regarding the treatment and management of the patient.
- Progress and effectiveness of treatment can be monitored.

There are drawbacks, mainly technical in nature:

- Making the slides, although not difficult, requires some practice.
- A trained, experienced technician is required to process and read the slides.
- Specific laboratory equipment and facilities are required.

RULES FOR POSSIBLE OR CONFIRMED MALARIA CASES

- Any person who complains of symptoms, and is awaiting diagnosis and treatment, should be made to lie down in a protected, cool area.
- Treat symptoms with paracetemol (e.g. Panado): 2 tablets every 4 hours (max 8/day). Avoid anti-inflammatories (e.g. Voltaren, Brufen) as these can lead to kidney failure.
- A **RAPID MALARIA** test must be performed without delay.
- If possible, **BLOOD SMEARS** should be performed if a reliable laboratory is available.

If malaria is diagnosed or suspected

Estimate the severity of the symptoms, by ticking off against the following checklist:

- Impaired consciousness – drowsy to coma
- Jaundice (yellow eyes)
- Repeated vomiting
- Cold, clammy and weak (usually this means low blood pressure)
- Temp >39 °C
- Low blood sugar (<2.5 mmol/l on meter)
- Cough
- Pallor
- Dehydration – sunken eyes, loss of skin elasticity
- No or little urine production (<400 ml in 24 hours)
- Pregnancy
- Under 5 years old
- High level of parasites in blood (>3%) diagnosed on a slide

If any of the above signs are present, this is an emergency. This signifies **COMPLICATED** malaria and the patient must be taken to expert medical care immediately.

TREATMENT OPTIONS (UNCOMPLICATED OR INTERIM MANAGEMENT OF COMPLICATED MALARIA)

Remember, if the malaria is complicated, the person should be transported to a hospital with an intensive care unit as soon as possible. If possible, intravenous quinine should be started before moving the patient by ground or air ambulance.

- **Co-artemether (Coartem)**

  Adults: 4 tablets immediately, then 4 tablets after 8 hours; then 4 tablets 12 hourly for 4 doses. Take pills with food that contains oil e.g. chips, bread and butter. Not for use in pregnancy.
  OR

- **Quinine and doxycycline**

  Adults: Quinine 600 mg (2 tablets) three times daily for 5 days after food, doxycycline 100 mg twice daily for 5 days starting on day 3. If used in pregnancy, substitute doxycycline with clindamycin 300 mg thee times daily for 5 days.
  OR

- **Atovaquone/proguanil**

  Adults: 4 tablets daily for 3 days. Take pills with food that contains oil e.g. chips, bread and butter. Not for use in pregnancy.
  OR

- **Mefloquine**

  Adults 750 mg (3 pills) immediately, followed by 500 mg (2 pills) 12 hours later. Not for use in pregnancy.

- **Halofantrine** (mentioned because it is freely available in much of the developing world)

  This drug should not be used outside a hospital, as it may cause sudden fatal cardiac arrhythmias.

FOLLOW-UP

Following therapy, and within 48 hours, there should be a marked decrease in the parasite count on the blood smear, coupled with a reduction in temperature and other signs and symptoms e.g. vomiting and diarrhoea.

CHILDREN

Children under five are at increased risk of death or complication from malaria. High levels of suspicion must be maintained, and acted upon if malaria is suspected. Children may present only with fever and often have a dry cough. Malaria in children under five is always to be regarded as complicated – but signs of dangerous malaria in children include:

- Confusion, drowsiness and delirium
- Seizures or convulsions
- Vomiting and diarrhoea
- Persistent cough with rapid respiration
- Pallor
- Jaundice

Treatment utilised may include the drugs as mentioned above in adults – except for Doxycycline in modified dosages.

TREATMENT FAILURE

A particular drug may fail because the parasites from a specific region may be resistant to the drug. The high likelihood of failure with chloroquine means that it is no longer a treatment option in most patients. Increasing resistance to Fansidar (sulphadoxine-pyrimethamine) may translate into treatment failure. Resistance to mefloquine is recorded, but is very infrequently seen, except for areas along the Thai-Myanmar (Burma) border.

It is usual to use another drug for treatment rather than the drug that has previously been taken in prophylactic form, e.g. if mefloquine was used as a prophylactic and taken conscientiously, and malaria still persists, it most likely means that the particular parasite is resistant to mefloquine.

Inadequate or insufficient earlier treatment may also result in a selection of parasites in a patient's body. If, for instance the malaria was treated with artemether alone, or another drug in insufficient dosage, the malaria would be controlled temporarily, but in a suppressed form. When it re-emerges, the active parasites are more likely to be those that survived the inadequate treatment by artemether. In that situation, an alternative drug is required.

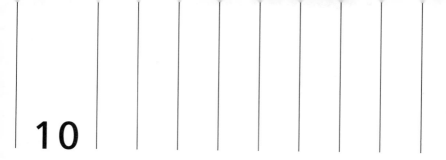

10

TESTING FOR MALARIA

WHAT SHOULD THE TEST SHOW THE DOCTOR?

Testing for malaria has been revolutionized in recent years by the introduction of rapid diagnostic tests, suitable for use both by doctors and laymen. These tests look for the presence in the patient's blood of proteins or 'antigens' derived from the malaria parasite. These tests are generally reliable and the newer ones will even differentiate infection with *P. falciparum* from the other malaria species. In most instances these tests will give an accurate result more than 80% of the time.

Rapid diagnostic tests resemble home pregnancy tests in both appearance and ease of use, generally comprising a paper strip onto which test chemicals have been impregnated, housed in a flat plastic case. A drop of the patient's blood is obtained and applied to the paper strip. If the test detects malaria, then at least two lines appear on the paper strip. If the test does not detect malaria, then a single 'control' line appears. Failure of the control line to appear indicates a defective test. Such a test would have to be discarded, and the test repeated with a fresh drop of blood and test strip.

Wherever possible, a positive rapid diagnostic test should be confirmed by microscopic examination of blood smears. The blood smears will not only confirm the diagnosis of malaria, but also reveal which species of *Plasmodium* is present, and the total percentage of red blood cells infected. A thick blood smear is examined to detect the presence of parasites, and a thin smear to determine the species. In many parts of the world, unfortunately, blood smear microscopy is not as reliable as it should be, and it is quite acceptable in such circumstances to base a diagnosis on a positive rapid diagnostic test alone.

In a non-immune person the percentage of red blood cells infected with malaria parasites gives an indication of the severity of the disease. A level of 1% is extremely worrying, while a parasite level of 5% or more may carry a grave prognosis.

In a person with some immunity, there is no absolute relationship between the number of parasites observed and the severity of the infection, as the person may be harbouring parasites in his blood without being symptomatic. However, if *P. falciparum* infection is suspected, treatment should proceed without waiting for confirmation.

A dangerous infection may be present in patients with a negative blood test result, especially when they have taken inadequate prophylactic antimalarial drugs or have been treated with some antibacterial agents or with antimalarials. The reason for this is that the drugs tend to mask the presence of the parasite in the blood, although the parasite infestation may still be low.

It is still a mystery among doctors that patients with heavy parasite infection can show few symptoms while those with low or undetectable parasites can manifest typical symptoms. Hence, although the test is very useful, it should not be relied upon absolutely when symptoms are otherwise indicative of malaria.

THE BEST TIME TO HAVE A TEST

The best time to have a test if malaria is suspected is immediately – do not wait for a fever spike.

WHEN WILL YOU GET THE RESULT?

Malaria results must be available within six hours. You should insist on being given the result; do not tolerate delays. It has happened in the past that malaria blood tests were treated as routine and only reported on three days later, with disastrous results.

TYPES OF TEST

Useful laboratory tests that the patient can ask the doctor for, include malaria parasite, platelet and white cell counts as well as measurements of haematocrit or haemoglobin, serum electrolytes and urea or creatinine. A request for liver function tests might also prove useful.

HOW ARE THE TESTS TAKEN?

Rapid malaria tests fall into two major types, depending on the technology used. The Parasight test uses a chemical found only in malaria parasites, and the others make use of an antigen detection mechanism. They are similar in their accuracy – around 80% – but are user dependant and people can make mistakes. Potential users should familiarise themselves with the techniques of testing while they are well, to avoid having to work it out from the start when feeling unwell. Remember, with all of these tests: if a control line is not seen, the test is not valid.

All tests naturally require a drop of blood, usually acquired by pricking a finger. Different tests vary a little in their exact method of employment, so be sure to read and follow the manufacturer's instructions. Follow the storage instructions too, to avoid being stuck with a dud test when you need it most.

Tests for microscopic examination require a technician to prick the patient's finger with a sterile lancet (see that the packet is opened in front of you). A thick blood smear is prepared by allowing a drop of blood to fall on a clean glass slide, which should then be allowed to dry before being stained and examined under the microscope. Thin smears are prepared in a similar way, with the drop of blood being spread across the glass slide.

Depending on which country you are in and on the facilities available, tests can take between 15 minutes to an hour before results are known. Every effort should be made to obtain test results as soon as possible because delay can prove fatal, especially if many hours have elapsed since the onset of malaria.

Worryingly, the reliability of microscopy in many developing countries is suboptimal, one American study finding local laboratories in some African countries reported smear results correctly only 25% of the time. Clearly, when travelling in developing countries, it would be unwise to accept a negative malaria test as conclusive proof that you do not have malaria, and smart to have your own rapid diagnostic kit available.

TAKING YOUR OWN TEST

If you are without virtually immediate access to reliable medical advice, you will have to take your own test. The rapid diagnostic tests are theoretically ideal for this, but the manufacturer's instructions must be followed scrupulously – studies have shown that inaccuracies in rapid diagnostic test results are mostly attributable to user error.

If you get a positive test result, then you should begin immediate treatment for malaria (see Appendix 1) and get yourself to a centre where reliable medical treatment is available, even if this means repatriation or evacuation. Initiating your own treatment might have come at a point in the disease's progress where complications are inevitable and skilled medical care essential.

WHAT TO DO WHEN TEST RESULTS ARE NEGATIVE AND YOU STILL SUSPECT YOU HAVE MALARIA

The general rule is to go ahead and treat for malaria if in any doubt at all. Once treatment is administered, parasites that are still in the blood will take two to three days to disappear so there is no point in testing after treatment unless you are using the Optimal test that becomes negative within a day or two of parasite elimination.

However, if after 48 hours symptoms are still being displayed, there is a strong chance that the treatment has not worked. At this point it is wise to have another test taken.

After adequate treatment the patient should be tested one to two weeks afterwards to confirm that parasites are not visible in the blood.

It must be noted that there is a difference between an infected person and a diseased person, as far as malaria is concerned. A person may be infected with the parasite and have it detectable in his blood, but due to semi-immunity, may not display any symptoms. The malaria parasite may be living in the person's blood, but it is not multiplying and causing problems – in many ways, it is benignly co-existing with the person. This contributes greatly to the spread of malaria in a community as these individuals are unaware of the malaria's presence in their blood, and do not seek treatment. On the other hand, a person may be infected and become diseased as a result of inadequate immunity. Hence those who are infected and become diseased are important links in the passing of the disease.

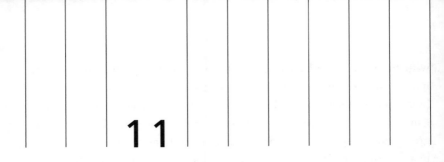

11

TREATMENT

THE MOST IMPORTANT ASPECTS OF TREATMENT
The following vital aspects of treatment cannot be stressed enough:
- prompt and effective treatment with antimalarials
- correction of fluid and electrolyte levels if there has been a fluid loss
- correction of hypoglycaemia or low blood sugar, especially in diabetics and pregnant women
- correction of anaemia
- treatment of concurrent infection if one exists

Bear in mind that statistics show that nearly all deaths in short-term travellers afflicted by malaria are caused by the lack of prompt and appropriate medical care.

WHEN TO TREAT FOR MALARIA
If *P. falciparum* is suspected, even if test results are not yet available or are negative, if the patient has fever or any of the other signs of malaria (see pages 38–41), an antimalarial treatment must be given. If another illness is suspected at the same time, treat for that as well.

The most important aim in treatment is to bring the level of parasites present in the blood under control as quickly as possible by the administration of rapidly acting drugs. This presents little difficulty, except in *P. falciparum* malaria where the progression of the disease is extremely rapid.

Because of the complicated nature of the drug treatment, the subject will be covered in Appendix 1. It is intended that in all cases where medical help is available, the patient should attempt to obtain it and not treat himself.

However, situations may arise where medical help is not available and a limited amount of information regarding the right and wrong drugs to take is likely to be better than no information at all.

Similarly, even where medical care is available, conflicting advice offered to the patient may cause him to wish to read his own information regarding drug treatment without having to seek out vast medical tomes in doing this research. This is where the information presented in the appendix is intended to assist the reader.

Information in Appendix 1 covers the different types of drugs available for the treatment of malaria, as well as side effects and contraindications. Suggestions are also made regarding complications such as how to treat fever, diarrhoea and vomiting.

12

THE COMPLICATIONS OF MALARIA

There are two directions malaria can take. One is uncomplicated malaria where aching joints, fever, headache and possibly nausea characterize the disease. All that needs to happen in this case is for the disease to be cured in time, either through medication or through the individual's own immune response if he has some immunity. In a person with no immunity, *P. falciparum* malaria will always progress and become life-threatening.

Malaria may present in its complicated form. Those listed below are all potentially serious and must be treated quickly and efficiently otherwise they may tip the balance towards death. It is important that the doctor treating the patient recognizes these complications as part of malaria and treats them accordingly.

VOMITING
This is a complication in the sense that it makes it impossible for necessary medication to be absorbed. Coupled with high fever, repeated vomiting also leads to dehydration (see pages 47–48). This complication develops especially rapidly in small children.

DIARRHOEA
This is characterized by the frequent passing of stools containing blood, mucous and blood cells. If not controlled, this condition can lead to potentially fatal dehydration, particularly if compounded by vomiting.

CHOLERAIC MALARIA

This is a condition in which profuse watery diarrhoea, nausea and vomiting occur. It is accompanied by muscular cramps, and the diarrhoea may be progressive. Dehydration is of major concern.

DEHYDRATION

Acute fever, vomiting, diarrhoea and anorexia all make dehydration worse. Adequate rehydration and the assurance of fluid intake are important determinants of clinical recovery, especially in young children. Failure to rehydrate may result in shock and kidney failure. Overhydration, especially with intravenous fluids, is equally dangerous and can be a factor in the development of major breathing problems.

JAUNDICE

This is a condition that must be monitored as it arises from the destruction of red blood cells by the malaria parasites. The remains of the destroyed blood cells collect in the body faster than they can be removed by the body's cleansing organs – the liver and the spleen.

One of the excess waste products is bilirubin that stains the whites of the eyes and the skin (especially the palms of the hands) yellow and is passed out in the urine, giving the latter a brownish colour, sometimes even turning it black. The best way to treat this kind of jaundice is to treat the malaria.

ENLARGEMENT OF THE SPLEEN

Like the liver, the spleen acts as a blood filter and when malaria strikes, it works overtime to clear the destroyed blood cells in the blood. Repeated exposure to malaria and thus a regular, heavy workload for the spleen results in enlargement and hardening that is especially palpable in young children. The fact that it is enlarged is not bad in itself and it usually subsides after effective treatment. The enlargement is thought not to affect the future workings of the spleen.

ACUTE KIDNEY FAILURE

Acute kidney failure may occur with *P. falciparum* malaria. The clinical features include confusion, restlessness, incoherence, jaundice and fever as well as decreased urine output.

It can be counteracted with adequate malaria treatment. The patient may need to be put on a dialysis machine. It is difficult to predict which cases of *P. falciparum* malaria will result in acute kidney failure.

ADVERSE DRUG INTERACTIONS

If you have been treated unsuccessfully and you then go to a different doctor for more treatment, toxic reactions may arise from adverse drug interactions, possibly leading to further delay in appropriate treatment and on the whole complicating the possibility of a positive outcome.

ACUTE RESPIRATORY DISTRESS SYNDROME (PULMONARY OEDEMA)

This may be caused by careless intravenous rehydration during severe *P. falciparum* infection. However, it may also arise before intravenous therapy has commenced. In many cases the patient needs to be put on a respirator until it improves.

CEREBRAL MALARIA

Cerebral malaria must be seen as an emergency, as once a coma sets in, deterioration is very rapid and the patient may die before intravenous drips can be set up (see section on cerebral malaria, pages 84–86).

BLACKWATER FEVER

This formerly common and extremely dangerous complication involves the presence of broken up blood cells in the urine, hence its name. It is associated with endemic *P. falciparum* malaria and is most often found in non-immune residents of malarious areas who have had a history of repeated clinical attacks that have been inadequately treated or suppressed by quinine. Cases can range from mild to severe with recovery quite possible in the milder cases.

The person who is more likely to suffer from blackwater fever tends to be in a state of hypersensitivity brought on by the presence of incompletely suppressed *P. falciparum* malaria. This syndrome may be triggered by a chill, exhaustion or injury.

It is an illness that is rarely seen these days. The literature seems to point to a link between inadequate administration and of quinine as a prophylactic in the days before synthetic antimalarials were available. This would seemingly explain why there was a much greater incidence of blackwater fever in days gone by.

CONVULSIONS

If a child is prone to convulsions, and malaria is suspected, the doctor must be informed. On the other hand if the child is not prone to convulsions, it should still be borne in mind that convulsions could occur especially in high levels of fever. They are also a feature of cerebral malaria.

ANAEMIA

Anaemia is an inevitable result of malaria and its severity is proportional to the intensity of the infection.

In some areas, many patients, particularly children, are already anaemic from other causes or from repeated previous attacks of malaria even before they develop severe malaria. This may be alleviated by blood transfusion, although in areas where blood is not routinely screened for HIV, this procedure can be risky.

A known blood donor should rather be sought, if possible, and appropriate measures should be taken to avoid over-transfusion.

Severe anaemia is a life-threatening complication. Treatment comprises rapid and effective clearance of parasites and transfusion where necessary. A particular trap is that these children may appear quite well, and chloroquine may be prescribed. Widespread resistance to chloroquine means that it can no longer be relied upon to give a cure, but despite this it is often prescribed in the developing world. Children treated with chloroquine in this situation may deteriorate disastrously with fatal consequences.

HYPOGLYCAEMIA (LOW BLOOD SUGAR)

Hypoglycaemia can be a complication in patients who are given quinine or quinidine intravenously or intramuscularly. It is most grave in pregnant women, a group that seems to be prone to low blood sugar.

Another high risk group is young children with severe malaria disease.

As hypoglycaemia may be confused with other symptoms and signs of severe malaria, blood glucose must frequently be checked, especially in the high-risk groups. It is also a frequent complication in African children.

Hypoglycaemia requires immediate specific treatment to prevent permanent brain damage. It causes confusion, coma and convulsions that closely resemble cerebral malaria. Treatment is intravenous using a concentrated sugar solution until the patient can take fluid and foods by mouth.

Blood glucose must be measured on admission and regularly thereafter in any child with any feature of severe malaria and in all pregnant women with malaria. In the absence of a means of testing blood sugar, hypoglycaemia should be assumed in any comatose child with malaria treated appropriately. Treatment with quinine may worsen the risk of low blood sugar.

SHOCK

This condition is characterized by vascular collapse and extreme coldness of the surface of the body. The temperature is subnormal and the blood pressure is low. If untreated the condition is fatal.

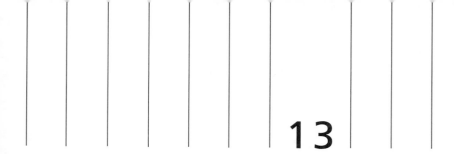

13

MALARIA IN PREGNANCY

Pregnant women should avoid going into malarious areas if at all possible. If this really is unavoidable, they should diligently guard against being bitten by mosquitoes, and must take appropriate prophylaxis. They should seek immediate medical help if any illness is suspected.

Complications in pregnancy such as miscarriage and stillbirth as well as death of the newborn are greatly enhanced by the infection of the mother and contribute to high maternal death rates in tropical malarious areas.

It is extremely important that medical help should be sought immediately malaria is suspected and treatment with an effective antimalarial must always be given.

Avoiding mosquito bites is always prudent, pregnant or not. Use of bednets, mosquito coils and window screens, the elimination of domestic breeding sites and going indoors after dusk can considerably lessen exposure.

Table 3: Advice to be given by prescribers to pregnant women and women of childbearing potential

Pregnant women

1. Malaria in a pregnant woman increases the risk of maternal death, neonatal death, miscarriage and stillbirth.
2. Do not go to a malarious area unless absolutely necessary.
3. Be extra diligent in the use of measures to protect against mosquito bites.

continued ...

4. Mefloquine (Lariam, Mefliam, Mephaquin) is now known to be safe in the second and third trimester of pregnancy. Despite limited experience, it is also believed by most experts to be safe in the first trimester as well.

5. Chloroquine and proguanil are considered to offer significantly less protection than mefloquine. In cases where proguanil (Paludrine) is used by a pregnant woman, she should also take folic acid supplements.

6. Doxycycline (Vibramycin and many other brands) is contra-indicated in pregnancy.

7. Seek medical help immediately if malaria is suspected, and take the emergency standby treatment (quinine is the drug of choice) only if no medical help is immediately available. Medical help must be sought as soon as possible after standby treatment.

Non-pregnant women of childbearing age

1. No harmful effects on the baby have been observed in the thousands of women who have fallen pregnant while taking mefloquine (Lariam, Mefliam, Mephaquin), despite earlier worries. It is no longer considered necessary to avoid pregnancy for three months after taking mefloquine.

2. Doxycycline (Vibramycin and many other brands) prophylaxis may be taken, but it may render the oral contraceptive pill less effective. Pregnancy should be avoided for about one week after stopping the drug.

3. If pregnancy occurs during antimalarial prophylaxis, except with chloroquine and proguanil (Paludrine) or with mefloquine (Lariam, Mefliam, Mephaquin), then information about the risks should be sought from the drug manufacturers by the woman's doctor.

(Extracted from the WHO *International Travel and Health Vaccination Requirements and Health Advice*)

WHAT ARE THE RISKS OF GETTING MALARIA IN PREGNANCY?

Pregnant women are more attractive to mosquitoes, so extra care should be taken to prevent bites, and they are more likely to contract malaria infections than women who are not pregnant, despite the fact that they may be resistant to the malaria parasite. Moreover, if and when they do become infected, they will display a higher parasite count in their blood.

Lowered resistance or increased vulnerability

Pregnancy reduces a mother's resistance to malaria, especially in early pregnancy. This vulnerability slowly reduces after the 24th week.

Of course, the non-immune mother who is, for instance, newly arrived in an endemic area, will be as vulnerable as any non-resistant person. However, pregnancy will complicate malaria and its treatment, should she contract it. This is why women who are pregnant or who are planning to become pregnant, are advised not to visit endemic countries.

In some circumstances, *P. falciparum* infection may be more severe during pregnancy, as a result of depressed maternal immunity. The risk of severe or fatal disease is greatest for the presumably resistant mother in areas of unstable transmission, where malaria is not transmitted year round, but only when conditions are favourable, such as during the rainy or hotter periods.

In contrast, pregnant women in areas of Africa with highly endemic malaria are generally not at greater risk of severe disease, particularly among women who are pregnant for the first time and who suffer from anaemia and the various complications of chronic parasite infection.

Risks during a first pregnancy

A woman pregnant for the first time is more likely to develop malaria than she will in later pregnancies. If a woman does develop malaria during her first pregnancy, she seems to develop some protection against malaria in her later pregnancies.

Malaria is particularly damaging to pregnant women during their first and second gestations when it can damage the foetus. A woman in her first pregnancy should therefore be especially alert for malarial symptoms and signs of possible complications and seek treatment promptly.

WHAT ARE THE SIDE EFFECTS OF MALARIA IN PREGNANCY?

P. falciparum malaria during pregnancy poses a threat to the life of the mother and the foetus and may lead to severe anaemia and foetal growth retardation. The impact of malaria during pregnancy on later development during infancy and childhood is not known.

Anaemia caused by malaria in pregnancy

Anaemia in pregnancy can cause foetal death, intrauterine growth retardation, low birth weight and premature delivery. Women who are pregnant for the first time and in their third trimester are at particular risk of severe anaemia and sometimes even death.

Anaemia among mothers who contract malaria is most common between the 16th and the 24th weeks and occurs when malaria parasites destroy red blood cells. Treatment of malaria in early pregnancy, when the mother's resistance is lowest, can prevent development of anaemia later in pregnancy. Iron or folic acid is of little benefit to the mother if malaria parasites continue to destroy red blood cells. Severe anaemia is aggravated by loss of blood during delivery.

Transplacental infection of the foetus

Premature or false labour is common in mothers infected with malaria. It is possible for the malaria parasite to infect the foetus via the placenta, resulting in the infant being born with malaria.

Transplacental infection of the foetus is far more common in non-immune mothers than in indigenous populations in malarious areas. A relationship exists between low birth weight and malarial infection of the placenta.

Although it may seem innocuous, low birth weight is an unnecessary handicap for an infant who may have to fight other handicaps at birth, such as jaundice or respiratory problems. Depending on the circumstances and neo-natal equipment available, the infant's chance of survival may be severely threatened.

Triggering a latent infection

The stress of childbirth may awaken a latent malaria infection in the semi-immune mother. Although her body may have kept the infection under control during pregnancy, the birth process may trigger the infection to the point where her body can no longer fight it and full-blown malaria develops. Either rapid treatment of acute infection or effective prophylaxis is therefore essential to avoid severe manifestations and complications.

TREATMENT OF MALARIA IN PREGNANCY

The consensus of medical opinion among malaria experts is that pregnant women who insist on visiting malarious areas should be protected with the most effective prophylaxis possible. Mefloquine (Lariam, Mefliam, Mephaquin) has been shown to be an effective and safe prophylactic during the second and third trimesters of pregnancy. There is less experience with the use of mefloquine in the first trimester, but the limited evidence available points to the drug being safe. Treatment of malaria must not be withheld during pregnancy and pregnant women in malarious areas should be protected by effective chemoprophylaxis during their pregnancy.

Earlier concerns that quinine may stimulate the pregnant uterus and induce abortion have been shown to be completely unfounded with the doses used to treat malaria. A pregnant woman diagnosed with malaria can and should receive immediate treatment with quinine.

Monitoring blood glucose

Monitoring of blood glucose by repeated finger-prick testing with indicator sticks is essential in pregnant women with malaria, especially if they are receiving intravenous doses of quinine, as they are more likely than other adults to develop hypoglycaemia or shortage of blood sugar. If they are at all able to eat or drink, it is preferable to try quinine by capsule or tablet rather than through a drip. Consider sugar supplementation in the diet, or in the intravenous fluid to prevent low blood sugar developing.

P. falciparum malaria in the third trimester in non-immune women has a poor prognosis. Fever and hypoglycaemia in the mother may cause foetal distress. As the lives of the mother and foetus may be at risk, obstetrical advice should be obtained about possible induction of labour, the speeding up of the second stage of labour with forceps or a vacuum extractor and even Caesarean section.

Antimalarial chemotherapy for pregnant women
It is generally agreed that prophylaxis in pregnancy is an effective strategy. A pregnant woman should research which drugs are safe and effective in her region and monitor changes in their efficacy. She must know the possible consequences of malaria and what to do if symptoms develop. In malarious areas it is recommended that all pregnant women receive rapid treatment for acute infection and effective prophylaxis, to avoid severe manifestations and complications (see also page 64). Intermittent presumptive treatment has been used in pregnant women in high risk areas, involving repeated and regular treatment for malaria throughout the pregnancy, without testing.

Chloroquine and quinine
Chloroquine and quinine have proved to be safe when used in normal therapeutic doses during pregnancy. Chloroquine may also be used prophylactically where it is effective.

Mefloquine (Lariam, Mefliam, Mephaquin)
Mefloquine is highly effective for the prophylaxis of malaria. Earlier concerns that it might be harmful to the foetus have proved unfounded, and it is known to be safe in the second and third trimesters. Limited experience with its use in

the first trimester has failed to reveal any harmful effects. It is regarded by most experts as the agent of choice for pregnant women visiting malarious areas.

Proguanil (Paludrine), chlorproguanil (Lapudrine) and dapsone-pyrimethamine (Maloprim)

The use of proguanil (Paludrine), chlorproguanil (Lapudrine) and dapsone-pyrimethamine (Maloprim) to prevent malaria in pregnancy continues in some countries. Widespread resistance to these drugs makes them a poor choice in most regions, however, and their use is best avoided unless no other drug is suitable. Dapsone-pyrimethamine (Maloprim) should be avoided in the third trimester. If proguanil (Paludrine) or dapsone-pyrimethamine (Maloprim) is used during pregnancy, a folic acid supplement is recommended.

Doxycycline (Vibramycin)

Doxycycline (Vibramycin) is contraindicated in pregnant women and in breastfeeding mothers.

TREATMENT OF ACUTE MALARIAL ATTACK IN PREGNANCY
A safe, universally acceptable treatment for malaria in pregnancy is not available. This is because all the treatment drugs carry the risk of certain side effects, depending on the individual's constitution. However, the following drugs have been used successfully.

Quinine

Quinine is accepted as both a safe and effective treatment for malaria in pregnancy, and is the treatment of choice. It is usually followed by a course of sulphadoxine-pyrimethamine (not in third trimester) or clindamycin to reduce the chances of quinine-resistant parasites emerging. Both malaria and the administration of quinine can cause increased insulin production leading to hypoglycaemia, which needs to be carefully monitored.

Mefloquine (Lariam, Mefliam, Mephaquin)

Although safe in pregnancy when used at prophylactic doses, concerns have been expressed about the safety of this drug in pregnancy when used in higher curative doses. Reports seem to indicate that women who receive this drug for treatment, as opposed to prophylaxis, are more likely to miscarry.

Sulphadoxine-pyrimethamine (Fansidar)

This drug is used in pregnancy, but principally for treatment of semi-immune residents of malarious areas. Increasing resistance is emerging.

Chloroquine

Although considered a safe drug in pregnancy, widespread resistance means that chloroquine should no longer be used to treat *falciparum* malaria. The consequences of treatment failure in pregnancy are too serious to justify the use of any but the most effective drugs.

Others

Other drugs have either not been proved safe in pregnancy, or have not proved themselves sufficiently effective to warrant recommendation. The first line of treatment in pregnancy remains quinine.

CHEMOPROPHYLAXIS, TREATMENT AND INFERTILITY

No specific link has been established between the taking of prophylactic and treatment drugs, but there is reason to believe that dapsone-pyrimethamine (Maloprim) and sulphadoxine-pyrimethamine (Fansidar) might reduce male fertility. If you are having problems with fertility, you should seek expert advice and question whether any drugs that you might be taking could interfere with fertility.

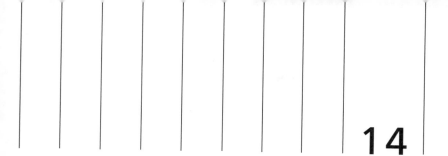

14

CHILDREN — AT SPECIAL RISK

Infants and young children can become seriously ill with malaria and are at special risk. If at all possible, they should not be taken to a malarial area. If unavoidable, then all measures possible must be taken to prevent them from being bitten by mosquitoes.

To be absolutely safe, fever in a child returning from a malarious area should be considered to be caused by malaria unless proved otherwise (according to the WHO).

INFANTS UP TO SIX MONTHS

When a pregnant woman is immune, a degree of immunity is conferred on the foetus from her across the placenta and such immunity is effective for approximately three to six months. Those infants with non-immune mothers are not likely to receive any immunity.

Natural immunity passes through the mother's breast milk to some extent but this has not been quantified. Infants may still become infected with malaria but seem to be resistant to developing cerebral malaria. They do become quite anaemic, however.

Even if the breast-feeding mother is taking prophylaxis herself, the amount of drug that passes through the breast milk is insufficient to bestow protection. It is therefore recommended that prophylaxis be given to breast-fed and bottle-fed infants.

Table 4: Advice to be given by prescribers to the parents

1. Children are at special risk since they can rapidly become seriously ill with malaria.

2. Do not take babies or children under the age of five years to a malarious area unless absolutely necessary.

3. Protect children against mosquito bites. Mosquito nets for cots and small beds are available. Keep babies under mosquito nets between dusk and dawn.

4. Give prophylaxis to breast-fed as well as bottle-fed babies, since they are not protected by their mother's prophylaxis.

5. Chloroquine and proguanil (Paludrine) may be given safely to babies and young children, but are no longer considered to offer the best protection available. For administration, drugs may be crushed and mixed with jam.

6. Where the package insert and manufacturer's directions are not available, calculate the antimalarial dose as a fraction of the adult dose based on the weight of the child.

7. Do not give sulphadoxine-pyrimethamine (Fansidar) or sulphalene-pyrimethamine or pyrimethamine and chloroquine (Daraclor) to babies under two months of age.

8. Mefloquine (Lariam, Mefliam, Mephaquin) may be given to infants of 5 kg weight or more, and is generally well tolerated by children.

9. Do not give doxycycline (Vibramycin) prophylaxis to children under 12 years of age.

10. Keep all antimalarial drugs out of reach of children and store in childproof containers. Chloroquine is particularly toxic to children if the recommended dose is exceeded.

11. Seek medical help immediately if a child develops a febrile (fever) illness. The symptoms of malaria in children may not be typical and so malaria should always be suspected. In babies less than three months old, malaria should always be suspected even in non-febrile illness.

(Extracted from the WHO *International Travel and Health Vaccination Requirements and Health Advice*)

SEVEN MONTHS TO FIVE YEARS

This is the most vulnerable period in a child's life when living in an endemic area on a long-term basis. The child can be compared, in terms of susceptibility, to a traveller who visits the area for the first time.

The child has to build up its own immunity and this is acquired over a long period of time during which the child keeps on getting bitten, and slowly raises its immunity.

The problem is that at the time of the first attack, which is likely to be the worst, the child still has minimal defences and is likely to die very quickly. Rapid diagnosis and treatment are of the utmost importance.

Attacks in endemic areas usually peak at about the age of two. Enlargement of the spleen often occurs as a result.

SIX TO 18 YEARS

By now a child living in an endemic area has built up a healthy immunity to malaria. Of course, infection by a parasite to which he is not immune can still cause severe illness and even death.

Note that a child in this age group, and indeed an adult, who arrives in an endemic area for the first time, is just as vulnerable as an infant or toddler and has to go through the same process of frequent bites over a reasonably long period in order to acquire immunity. It is worth investigating which treatment drugs will work in the malarious area you will be visiting or living in (with some drugs now becoming available in suppository form).

It is not known why certain people, having lived in an endemic area for years, without taking prophylaxis, and without even getting malaria, finally get it, and get it very severely.

SYMPTOMS IN CHILDREN

Confusingly, many children with very high parasite densities in the bloodstream often display fairly mild symptoms. Therefore, the highest suspicion of malaria should be regarded in a serious light and efforts should be made to have the child's blood tested for diagnosis.

In children the manifestations are often atypical and may be alarming. Paroxysms of fever are less common, while headache, nausea, vomiting, abdominal pain, diarrhoea, a sustained fever and convulsions make up a much less characteristic clinical picture.

CEREBRAL MALARIA IN CHILDREN

Despite optimal care, between 10% and 30% of children suffering from cerebral malaria die.

This condition is frequently the only manifestation of severe *P. falciparum* infection in children. Convulsions form part of the symptoms of cerebral malaria.

DIAGNOSIS

P. falciparum is usually very severe in children from non-endemic areas; diagnosis may be difficult, because parasites may not be found easily, and multiple blood smears may be taken if the first are negative. If the child is on prophylaxis and the blood smear is negative, a careful judgement, taking into account the type of prophylaxis taken, active strains in the area and severity of illness, should be made before deciding to treat for malaria.

The incubation period is usually from six to 15 days and there are no distinctive signs in this period that the child may have contracted malaria. The first signs that he may have malaria are listlessness, restlessness and drowsiness; he may refuse food and there may be headaches or nausea. Fever is usual but variable and irregular; a regular fever cycle is uncommon and therefore not reliable as a symptom of malaria. Diarrhoea may occur and a dry cough is common. The spleen enlarges and is tender, but diagnosis should not depend on this.

Some children in highly endemic areas acquire a relative tolerance to the infection and suffer only a mild illness. Many children in such areas have large livers and spleens and malaria parasites in the blood, but no other signs of the disease.

HOW MUCH TIME DO YOU HAVE WITH CHILDREN?

Life-threatening complications may develop very rapidly in children with malaria. That is why time is so important in the treatment of the disease. In children the interval between the onset of symptoms and death may be about 48 hours, although cases have occurred where death results only after a few hours.

CHEMOPROPHYLAXIS

A distinction must be made between residents of an endemic area who will live there all their lives, and those, such as expatriates, who eventually intend leaving the area.

Chemoprophylaxis is strongly indicated for non-local children who have not had frequent exposure to bites over a long period. It has not been established what effect long-term prophylaxis will have on a child's development, although there is no evidence that long-term prophylaxis is harmful. What is known is that children experiencing repeated bouts of malaria are likely to suffer decreased cognitive ability and delayed mental development.

It is important to remember that if a child is taken out of the endemic area for any length of time, say for a three-month holiday, his levels of immunity will drop during the time he is away and his vulnerability will be increased when he returns to the endemic area. This is because immunity is dependent on frequent exposure to mosquito bites and infection.

- Chloroquine and pyrimethamine should not be given to infants younger than six weeks.
- Proguanil (Paludrine) may be safely given to babies and young children. It may be combined with chloroquine in infants older than six weeks.
- Doxycycline (Vibramycin) is not recommended for children under the age of 12 years.
- Mefloquine (Lariam, Mefliam, Mephaquin) should not be given to children weighing less than 5 kg.

ADMINISTRATION OF ANTIMALARIALS TO CHILDREN

The administration of bitter drugs like mefloquine (Lariam, Mefliam, Mephaquin) to children is always difficult and there is no evidence that syrups are easier to administer than tablets crushed and mixed with water, jam or condensed milk. It may also help to control spillage if a 5 ml syringe is used to administer the drug.

Force is often necessary (including closing the child's nostrils to make him open his mouth). There is a risk of inhalation of the medicine. A certain quantity of the drug may be spat out, leading to underdosage – or even overdosage if repeated attempts are made to administer the drug.

Most studies suggest that as suppression of malaria by prophylaxis is never complete, exposure to parasites while under the relative protection of prophylaxis might stimulate the immune system to help maintain some level of actively acquired immunity.

SUGGESTED COURSE OF TREATMENT IF MALARIA IS SUSPECTED IN A CHILD

Paracetamol and liquids for children needing oral rehydration are administered immediately and the skin is cooled with tepid water and by fanning. After that a blood smear should be taken if possible. The result should be available in ten to 30 minutes.

The child may then be fit enough to take curative drugs orally if needed. If the child is not able to take medication by mouth he would have to be admitted to hospital and put on a drip. Artesunate is available for paediatric use in some countries in suppository form – this can be used in the presence of vomiting or an unco-operative child.

COMPLICATIONS IN THE TREATMENT OF CHILDREN

Vomiting may complicate the treatment of malaria, especially in children. When associated with a high fever, vomiting is frequently an indication for intravenous therapy, but experience shows that, in a substantial proportion of children with fever, oral therapy will be possible within one or two hours after a reduction of fever. (For more information, see also Chapter 12: Complications of malaria.)

THE LONG-TERM CONSEQUENCES OF MALARIA

Repeated malaria leads to severe anaemia that increases vulnerability to other diseases and hampers development. Of course, severe anaemia itself can quickly lead to death.

Recent studies of African children who have suffered repeated bouts of malaria show evidence of stunting of intellectual development and poor scholastic performance.

15

CEREBRAL MALARIA

Cerebral malaria can be defined as a state of altered consciousness in a patient who has *P. falciparum* parasites in the blood and in whom no other cause of altered consciousness can be found (according to the WHO). In children, cerebral malaria is frequently the only manifestation of severe *P. falciparum* malaria. Other strains of malaria, i.e. *P. ovale, P. malariae* and *P. vivax*, do not cause cerebral malaria.

It is not proved, but the symptoms are attributed to infected red cells clogging the inner lining of the capillaries of the brain. These infected red cells tend to become sticky and less flexible, causing a plugging or blocking effect, thus reducing the flow of circulation.

Contrary to popular belief, any form of *P. falciparum* can cause cerebral malaria. Certain individuals are more prone to this complication than others, but there is no practical way of predicting this.

DIAGNOSIS
Confusingly, many patients with cerebral malaria have scanty parasite counts and, conversely, many children with high parasite densities have fairly mild symptoms.

The longer the illness or resulting coma, the more likely the patient is to die or develop neurological complications, a wide range of which has been observed. These include cortical blindness, blindness on one side, motor disorders, spasticity and severe mental impairment.

The diagnosis of cerebral malaria is made clinically, but if there is any doubt about the diagnosis, then a lumbar puncture will most likely be recommended, to exclude bacterial meningitis or subarachnoid haemorrhage. In cerebral malaria the lumbar puncture usually reveals only minimal abnormalities, although raised intracranial pressure may be present. If the attending doctor is able to examine the back of the eye, the presence of tiny haemorrhages may alert him to the diagnosis of cerebral malaria.

SYMPTOMS

Adults with malaria commonly have problems in other organs, usually the lungs and the kidneys.

Cerebral malaria develops very rapidly. Levels of consciousness can vary from mild confusion to deep coma.

The rapidity of the descent into unconsciousness and in survivors of the emergence into full awareness are unique, distinguishing and intriguing features of cerebral malaria.

The illness may start with increasing headache, restlessness or even bizarre behaviour in rare cases. A generalized convulsion is often followed by increasing drowsiness leading to stupor and coma.

Patients with cerebral malaria often have a shortage of blood sugar or glucose. Since this is important for the brain to function, the low sugar level may worsen an already poorly functioning brain.

In adults (except those with a history of epilepsy), convulsions are a sign of cerebral malaria. Convulsing carries a real risk of inhalation of stomach contents or vomit. This is an under-recorded cause of death in cerebral malaria.

TREATMENT

Treatment drugs of first choice are intravenous quinine or quinidine.

Prophylactic administration of phenobarbitone decreases the number of subsequent convulsions in adults and children with cerebral malaria who are already prone to convulsions.

Measures to reduce the likelihood of convulsions and their consequences should be rigorously applied: the temperature of children should be kept as close to normal as possible by sponging with tepid water and fanning and the regular, rather than intermittent, use of paracetamol.

Patients suffering from advanced cerebral malaria require the highest level of nursing care available as they are unconscious and liable to convulsions, vomiting, aspiration pneumonia and the complications of prolonged immobility.

PROGNOSIS

The majority of those dying from cerebral malaria are children under the age of five. The acute inflammation caused by cerebral malaria accounts for over 80% of deaths from malaria. Between 10% and 50% of people with cerebral malaria die. Survival depends on the level of care available and the age of the patient, among other things.

In those who survive, particularly children, recovery is surprisingly rapid. More than half recover in less than 24 hours while the rest recover in 24 to 48 hours.

The prognosis for cerebral malaria is positive, provided treatment is timely, apt and rapid. If the patient is reached before too much damage is done to the brain, then recovery will take place within 48 hours. It is, however, not uncommon for those who do recover from cerebral malaria to suffer from some type of neurological defect, although some people recover without any long-lasting negative effects.

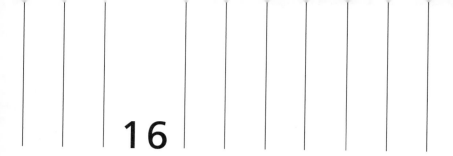

16

RECURRING MALARIA

Malaria may recur months or even years after apparent successful treatment. In patients infected with *P. vivax* or *P. ovale*, this phenomenon is known as relapse.

Relapse is caused by dormant liver stage forms of the parasite, which resume their development cycle and release merozoites back into the bloodstream.

THE DIFFERENCE BETWEEN RELAPSE AND RECRUDESCENCE

It is a common misconception that all types of malaria are liable to relapse. This is not true as *P. falciparum* will only recrudesce if treated incorrectly or insufficiently and the period of recurrence is limited to under a year, while the other types of malaria will cause relapse even if they are 'cured'. We can now, by examining the genetic makeup of the malaria parasite, determine whether the infection is a new one or one that was incurred previously.

The recurrence of malaria caused by *P. falciparum* and *P. malariae* is due to a break-through caused by surviving blood-stage parasites from an earlier infection. In the case of *P. falciparum,* break-throughs usually occur within a matter of weeks rather than months. In other strains, recurrence can be interrupted by long periods of dormancy of the parasite.

P. falciparum infections will not recur provided that prophylactic and treatment dosages have been taken correctly as prescribed (taking into account possible resistance) and provided that the strain of parasite is sensitive to the drug used.

In untreated or inadequately treated malaria, the parasite may persist in the body for months or years.

After the early period of recurring fever (overt malaria), the parasites are more or less in equilibrium with the forces of immunity. It is not known what triggers the sudden increase in growth in the parasites.

P. vivax malaria is characterized by a tendency to relapse from the dormant liver stage and, even if a suitable prophylactic drug has been taken regularly and continued for one month after the last risk of exposure to infection, such relapses may occur (unless a course of primaquine has been taken) and have been known to do so up to 13 months after the prophylactic was discontinued.

This may cause difficulty in diagnosis. It is recommended that anti-relapse treatment of *P. vivax* infections with primaquine should be limited to two categories of patients: those living in areas where there is no *vivax* present or areas with low levels of transmission, and those leaving the malarious area.

It is not necessary to provide anti-relapse treatment routinely to a patient living in an endemic area; in case of relapse or reinfection, such patients should be treated with an effective drug such as chloroquine. It is a good idea for long-term expatriate travellers to have their blood G-6-P-D level tested before departure, to enable them to be treated with a drug such as primaquine, should it become necessary. This test can be difficult to obtain in the developing world.

17

CHRONIC MALARIA

The term 'chronic' is applied to repeated reinfections as a result of either inadequate prophylaxis or treatment.

Chronic malaria causes progressive enlargement of the spleen, which acts as a blood-cleansing organ and supplier of malaria antibodies. It is overtaxed in those who have suffered regular malaria attacks and hence becomes enlarged. This is particularly noticeable in children.

In some adults who are infected with malaria, the body seems to lose control over the spleen, which continues to enlarge and eventually becomes extremely large. This condition often requires long-term antimalarial treatment. Surgical removal of the spleen is not advised.

The liver also becomes enlarged and firm, and biochemical tests may reveal a certain amount of liver dysfunction.

Children who suffer from frequent attacks of malaria do not thrive. These repeated malaria attacks deplete the body and also produce anaemia that further weakens the system. Malaria is probably a causative factor of stunted growth.

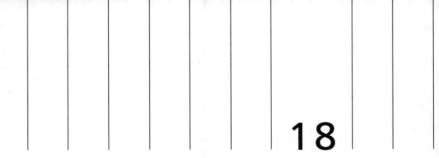

18

MIXED INFECTIONS

Mixed infections are fairly common and result when two mosquitoes carrying two different species of the malaria parasite bite a person within a short space of time. It is also possible that one mosquito can carry two different parasites and infect the victim with both when taking its blood-feed.

Thus two different infections develop independently. During diagnosis, with blood smears, the technician is likely to notice the dominant infection and therefore reporting of mixed infections is not as common as it might be.

The possibility of whether a mixed infection compounds the illness has not been well studied.

In terms of treatment, medication prescribed to treat *P. falciparum* will be effective against other species. A course of primaquine will need to follow the acute stage treatment to eliminate the relapsing malarias, however.

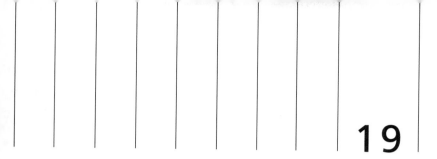

19

HOW IMMUNITY AFFECTS YOUR RESPONSE TO MALARIA

THE DEFINITION OF IMMUNITY

Immunity may be natural or acquired, and complete or partial. Over many centuries those who were highly vulnerable to malaria died off, while the surviving members of the population were naturally selected from stock that possessed a high natural immunity to the disease.

It is interesting to note tht some Africans possess an inherited trait that protects them from malaria: in this condition, called sickle cell anaemia, the haemoglobin is abnormal.

Generally, human immunity to the disease results from a capacity, following ancestral exposure to malaria, to produce proteins that specifically neutralize the harmful effects of the infecting organism. Of the two types of immunity – natural immunity (genetic/inherited) or acquired immunity, neither gives complete protection against attacks.

THE ERADICATION OF MOSQUITOES AND THE LOSS OF IMMUNITY

Ironically, it appears that the eradication of mosquitoes from a malarial area might in the long run backfire on the immune inhabitants. In time, they would inevitably lose their immunity and the chance reintroduction of infected mosquitoes to their countries from another area would result in devastating epidemics.

PREGNANCY AND IMMUNITY

In pregnancy, a degree of immunity from the already immune mother is transferred via the placenta, causing the infant to remain immune for the first three to six months of life.

DIFFERING DEGREES OF IMMUNITY

It is thought that immunity may come in different degrees, for example, delay in development of the infection, mild parasitaemia (parasite counts) and complete resistance.

HOW IMMUNITY IS BUILT UP

Immunity is built up slowly and over time. It is acquired by repeated bites from malaria-carrying mosquitoes.

A person acquires his own immunity to malaria when he has been living within a malaria-endemic area for a fair length of time, a period that is closely related to the amount of exposure he has had to the bites of infected mosquitoes. It is unusual for an adult who moves into a region to develop any significant semi-immunity at all. Furthermore, should an adult who has grown up in a region, leave that region for more than a year, any semi-immunity will in all likelihood be severely reduced or lost. Returning nationals going home to visit friends and relatives should be aware that they should regard themselves as non-immune 'foreigners', with all the attendant risks of developing severe malaria.

It is not known exactly why a person does not get full-blown malaria each time he is bitten by an infected mosquito. It is thought that each dose is small enough for the body's immune system to cope with and overcome, but this has not been proved.

SPECIFIC IMMUNITY

If the first five years of childhood are successfully negotiated, a balance is achieved between infection and resistance.

Resistance is developed against the specific strain of malaria a person is most exposed to. Therefore, if you move to a different part of the country and are infected by a different strain there, your immune system may not be able to recognize and fight that particular strain.

TYPES OF IMMUNITY

As immunity is rarely complete, long-term residents of malarious areas may at best be regarded as being partially or semi-immune:

- *non-immune* e.g. travellers, young children, military personnel, refugees, tourists and those in whom established immunity has lapsed, pregnant women (who are more vulnerable), inhabitants of an endemic area who leave and then return and residents of an area where a successful malaria control programme has been concluded.
- *partially or semi-immune* e.g. those who live in areas where transmission of malaria is irregular, for instance only during the rainy season; or those who spend a fair amount of time outside their country of residence where transmission is year-round. Long-term residents who remain continuously in malarious areas will eventually develop higher levels of immunity, but may nevertheless still be prone to infection. Those who live continually in a country where malaria transmission is year-round and who have lived their childhood years in the same place are likely to develop reasonable levels of resistance.

Non-immune

If travel to malarious areas is unavoidable, prior to departure travellers should obtain the address of reliable medical services at their destination, and ensure that they have insurance for emergency evacuation to their home country.

If the traveller is likely to be hypersensitive to an antimalarial drug or is taking other drugs for long-term medical conditions, he should consult a doctor with specialized knowledge of the problem before departure and decide whether his journey is essential.

The traveller who is lacking a spleen, has problems with his immune system, or suffers from diseases such as lymphoma, cardiac conditions, leukaemia (even in remission) or Hodgkin's disease, should make prior arrangements for adequate medical care at his destination and should seek this care immediately if he should fall ill.

It is generally recommended that women who are pregnant should not travel to malarious areas (see relevant section on pregnancy, pages 69–76). Pregnant women, as well as children under five years of age, are most vulnerable to contracting malaria. During pregnancy the immune system is not at its best. Expectant mothers exposed to malaria are most vulnerable during first or second pregnancies, and in the first trimester of pregnancy.

As the malignant malaria (*P. falciparum*) parasites take between six and 15 days to incubate, and those parasites responsible for the more benign forms (mainly *P. vivax*) may take much longer to incubate, a disease that starts before six days have elapsed since the first exposure is probably not malaria.

Early diagnosis and prompt treatment are the most vital survival tools for those who may have malignant malaria. A non-immune person who develops fever six days or more after the first possible exposure to malaria should seek prompt medical attention while informing the doctor that he may have malaria. Most travellers who contract malaria initially develop the disease without complications although the progression to severe anaemia is usually very rapid.

The choice of drug treatment for travellers (see Appendix 1, pages 111–129) depends, as it does with all malaria patients, on the species of malaria parasite prevalent where the infection was contracted. Parasite sensitivities to antimalarial drugs vary greatly around the world (see pages 22–29).

Depending on the country visited, the appropriate drugs and prompt medical attention may not be available. Non-immune travellers are advised to carry their own rapid diagnostic kits and appropriate antimalarial drugs for stand-by treatment. This stand-by treatment may be used as self-treatment but, preferably, should be used only after obtaining reliable medical advice.

Because of the possibility of toxic reactions, travellers should resort to self-treatment only if they have good reason to suspect malaria and prompt medical attention is not available.

Medical attention should be sought at the earliest possible opportunity and the doctor should be told which drugs were taken and in what dosages. If possible, keep a close watch on symptoms and note them down so that you can inform the doctor of the progression of the disease.

The typical symptoms of malaria are bouts of high fever lasting a few hours, beginning with shaking chills, subsiding with profuse sweating, and recurring at several intervals, usually every 48 hours.

It is worth noting that the signs are often atypical during the first few days and are less typical in malignant than in benign malaria.

Therefore the possibility of malaria should be considered in all otherwise unexplained fevers in non-immune persons who have been exposed to mosquitoes.

Semi-immune

Partial or semi-immunity develops over time through repeated infection and without recurrent infection. Immunity is relatively short-lived when malaria transmission is not ongoing in the country of residence or when the person has spent lengthy periods of time out of his country of residence, thereby losing any immunity he may have gained.

People with partial immunity may still contract malaria if they are exposed to strains of the parasite against which they have not developed immunity, or if their resistance is lowered through intercurrent illness or stress. There is reason to believe that Africa's HIV epidemic may amplify malaria transmission on the continent, as it will lower the resistance of millions of people.

There is really no such thing as a person who is fully immune to malaria. He may be almost completely immune to one or two strains of parasite but because of geographical variations in the distribution of the various strains of malaria parasite, he may not be immune to strains prevalent in areas that he rarely visits.

The mechanism by which the body's immune system fights off malaria is known to be extremely complex, but it is still incompletely understood. This partly explains why a malaria vaccine has been so long coming. It is known that the spleen plays a central role in immunity against malaria, and people without spleens are at high risk of death if they contract malaria.

People with high levels of immunity have lived in an area with year-round malaria transmission for a very long time, or they have an inherited tendency to overcome malaria.

If and when they do get malaria, it is generally not severe, although there are of course some cases that are, and the individual is usually able to overcome the infection on his own. There may be fever or vague complaints of headache, body pains or a general malaise.

Without repeated exposure however, this immunity is relatively short-lived and, although it almost always protects against life-threatening malaria, it does not prevent occasional bouts of fever and chills.

Researchers postulate that some people tolerate malaria infections without symptoms whereas others are severely affected because they have become sensitized to the breakdown products formed by the parasite.

PREVENTION OF RELAPSES

The drugs recommended for prophylaxis do not eliminate the liver stages of relapsing malaria infections i.e. *P. vivax* in most of the malarious areas and *P. ovale* in West Africa.

The liver stages can lead to relapses up to three years after exposure, but these relapses are not life-threatening.

These relapsing malarias can only be eliminated by primaquine, but anti-relapse courses are usually recommended only for persons with proven relapsing malaria. Primaquine should only be taken under medical supervision, and after a blood test to exclude G-6-P-D deficiency, an inherited disorder common in some ethnic groups.

20

HOW CAN YOU AVOID GETTING MALARIA?

Medical consensus is that malaria should be avoided at all costs. For this reason, personal protection measures to prevent mosquito bites and chemo-prophylaxis should both be used, as neither can be relied upon to provide complete protection. Neither should be neglected on account of the other.

In addition, protection largely depends on the individual's motivation to seek useful advice and act upon it. It depends on the perception of risk to which the person is exposed and the severity of malaria. The individual must also understand the types of protective measures that are at his disposal and his need to comply with these measures.

Most of the above conditions may be met, but if coupled with less than perfect compliance, especially with chemoprophylactic measures, then protection may be reduced significantly.

Among travellers, in particular, reasons for non-compliance include forgetfulness, especially by those who travel often and have busy schedules; inadequate information and time for preparation prior to departure; confusion from contradictory information; unpleasant side effects of the drug or other illness; or that recommended protective measures are complicated.

Those travelling to endemic areas where drug resistance is experienced should be made aware of the type of symptoms that may develop despite taking antimalarial drugs, and that may well indicate a malaria infection. They should realize that symptoms can become apparent while they are still in the area or even after they have stopped taking prophylaxis up to a period of three months after their return. They must also know what to do in the event that they experience symptoms.

Personal protection measures and protection through the use of prophylactic drugs should be individualized. The following factors should be taken into account when deciding what type of prophylaxis to take and what sort of personal protection measures to adopt:

- Prevalence of mosquitoes in area visited.

  Is it situated at high or low altitude?

  Is the area likely to be in city centres with air-conditioned buildings?

  Is the visit during the wet or dry season?

- Incidence of the parasite's resistance to the drug will determine which drugs are likely to confer protection.
- Purpose of visit (e.g. business or safari).
- Type of accommodation available (i.e. screened or air-conditioned).
- Duration of stay in the area – the longer the visit, the greater the risk of contracting malaria. Long-term prophylaxis has been shown to be safe in a number of good scientific studies.
- Time of year (is transmission steady throughout the year or are there peak periods of transmission?).
- Availability of drugs.
- Toxicity of the available drugs.
- Age of the patient, which will determine drug selection and dosage as well as vulnerability to malaria.
- Pregnancy or lactation.
- Immune status.
- Medical facilities and their availability and adequacy.
- Drug allergies.
- Concurrent medication and illnesses.
- Use of protective measures, their efficacy and compliance with them.

No prophylactic regimen can be expected to give perfect protection. To complicate matters, most drugs used for prophylaxis are associated with some toxic side effects.

Whatever preventive measures are adopted and prophylaxis taken, it is essential that they be backed up by prompt diagnosis and treatment of malaria.

In the light of the potentially fatal consequences of malaria, travellers at especially high risk, such as the very young and pregnant women, should consider very carefully whether travel to malarious areas is unavoidable. Other persons at high risk who should avoid a malarious area altogether are individuals whose immune systems are compromised i.e. those who are on long-term steroid therapy; cancer patients on chemotherapy; AIDS patients; and those who have had their spleens removed.

Measures that prevent infection involve personal protection against bites with mosquito coils, vapours, sprays and nets.

The only measure for protecting against disease without preventing infection would be immunisation, an option that will not be available to us for a long time yet.

21

MECHANICAL PROTECTION

International Travel and Health Vaccination Requirements and Health Advice, published by the WHO, includes the following guidelines:

- If available, choose screened or air-conditioned accommodation (remember: doors to such accommodation should be kept closed unless they are screened, to prevent the daily entry of mosquitoes).
- Where this is not available, make effective use of a mosquito net preferably impregnated with insecticide.
- Use long-sleeved clothing and trousers when outdoors in the evening; keep the ankles protected as much as possible.
- Apply a mosquito repellent to exposed skin (while taking note of manufacturer's recommendations, especially for young children).
- Where screened sleeping accommodation is available, clear the room of any resting mosquitoes by using an insecticide aerosol, preferably a synthetic pyrethroid.
- Where electricity is available, plug in insecticide dispensers using mats impregnated with synthetic pyrethroid. They are a compact and useful addition to the traveller's kit.
- Don't go outside at night if you can avoid it. Bear in mind that large numbers of indigenous children are usually carriers of malaria parasites; avoid staying nearby if possible.
- Don't allow children to play in dark, shady areas. Avoid places with banana, sisal and maize plantations nearby as they may provide resting sites for mosquitoes.

- Where safe sprays are available, it is advisable to spray the internal walls of houses every three months.
- All ventilation holes should be screened to prevent insects from coming through them.
- Make sure there are no containers of water exposed, in which mosquitoes can breed.
- Insecticide-impregnated mosquito nets have proved to be highly effective, but they must be scrupulously maintained to avoid tearing. There should be no opening on the side of the net, which ideally should be lowered and tucked well under the mattress before dusk and not raised until after dawn. Mosquitoes will enter a torn or sloppily used net, which then becomes a mosquito-trap.
- Long-term residents in malarious areas should, if they can, situate houses a kilometre or more away from water points or streams; hilltops are usually better than valleys. The windows of houses should be covered by special metal gauze manufactured for the purpose. Mosquito-proof screen doors may be added to outside doors so that they can be kept open to allow maximum air movement inside without letting mosquitoes in.
- Mosquitoes tend to lurk under tables and chairs and the ankles are therefore particularly vulnerable to bites. Two pairs of stockings are not enough to prevent bites.
- When spraying a room, pay particular attention to dark corners, spaces beneath chairs and tables and also to wardrobes, cupboards, bathrooms and lavatories.

22

QUESTIONS COMMONLY ASKED ABOUT MALARIA

Are the following statements true?

- If you habitually drink gin and tonic you are less likely to get malaria. (Answer: The level of quinine in the tonic is thought to be too low to prevent malaria.)
- If you are bitten in the afternoon, it will not be by a mosquito carrying the malaria parasite. (Answer: It is unlikely to be by one carrying malaria.)
- Only the female mosquito will transmit malaria. (Answer: Yes.)
- The malaria-carrying mosquito makes no noise. (Answer: It makes a slight noise.)
- If I have AIDS and get malaria, I will die from the attack. (Answer: Yes, unfortunately you are at risk of more serious malaria, and malaria may also make your HIV infection worse by increasing viral load.)
- Malaria will surface when the host's immune system is compromised. (Answer: Yes, unless there is a balance between immunity and parasite levels.)
- With *P. ovale* malaria, your body will have overcome the infection after three years. (Answer: Yes, as the parasite stops relapsing.)
- You can contract malaria from a blood transfusion. (Answer: Yes, if the blood has not been screened properly for malaria parasites.)
- Malaria can exist in cold climates such as England. (Answer: Whatever malaria exists will be short-lived and invariably brought over on an

aeroplane from a malarious country. The onset of cold weather usually prevents the extended propagation of the disease in countries with cooler climates. Should global warming become a reality, however, it is quite possible that some temperate regions may see a return of at least seasonal malaria.)

- There are long-term effects of malaria. (Answer: Yes; some victims report disturbing psychological symptoms, while children who suffer frequent attacks exhibit some dulling of intellect. Anaemia can also result when the ongoing destruction of the blood cells by maturing malaria parasites over a period of time gradually lowers the blood count; disturbed liver function and enlarged spleen are results of ongoing parasite infection.)

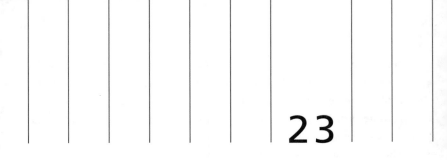

23

THE LONG-TERM OUTLOOK FOR MALARIA

WHAT DOES THE FUTURE HOLD?

Globally, the malaria situation is worsening. This is partly due to the complex nature of the malaria parasite, which has enabled it so successfully to resist the numerous and varied attempts to both control and eradicate it. It would also be fair to say that the current dire situation is also partly attributable to inadequate and half-hearted control measures, and improper drug use.

The current WHO-inspired Multilateral Initiative on Malaria and Roll Back Malaria campaigns aim to bring new and affordable drugs to the fight against malaria, and to reduce the total world burden of this disease by 50% by 2010.

The rapid rate at which the parasite develops drug resistance has led the WHO to set the goal of providing the world with at least one new antimalarial every five years, as prospects for the reversal of established drug resistance do not look good. Despite media hype to the contrary, the Holy Grail of an effective and dependable malaria vaccine suitable for mass use remains years away.

NEW DRUGS

Every so often, a so-called 'new' drug to treat or prevent malaria receives media attention. Sadly, most of these are really old drugs reformulated, usually in combination with another existing drug. Nevertheless, there have been some developments worthy of attention, and which do represent an advance, including some of the not really so novel 'new' drugs.

ARTEMESININ

Drug research has aroused much interest in artemesinin, a new class of antimalarial drug that has roots in ancient Chinese history.

For some 2 000 years, the leaves and flowering heads of *Artemisa annua* (the sweet wormwood plant) have been used in Chinese traditional medicine to treat the fever and chills associated with malaria. A range of drugs goes under the heading of 'artemesinins'. These drugs are all pretty similar and bear names showing their membership of the artemesinin group, e.g. artemether, artesunate.

Artemesinins have marked activity against malaria parasites, including multidrug-resistant *P. falciparum*. Available in oral, suppository, and intramuscular injection form, artemesinins are slowly gaining acceptance in the West, and have been licensed in a number of developed countries.

Artemesinin derivatives have been extensively studied. The results show that they are capable of rapid initial clearance of parasitaemia (within hours only), faster than any other drug, and that they are effective against *P. falciparum*. They are usually well tolerated, but may possess some neurotoxicity. However, malaria frequently recrudesces when treated with artemesinins alone, and these drugs must be used in combination.

When used in carefully selected combination (see Appendix 1 and below), artemesinins give speedy relief without recrudescence. They are best used for the treatment of uncomplicated malaria.

ARTEMESININ COMBINATIONS

Artemesinins have been successfully combined with mefloquine, and with another Chinese drug, benflumetol. The latter is also known as lumafantrine, and is related to halofantrine (Halfan). Unlike halofantrine, however, it has not demonstrated any worrying cardiac side effects, and it is considered to be relatively safe.

The combination of artemether and benflumetol is known as co-artemether (Co-Artem or Riamet). It is useful for the treatment of uncomplicated malaria.

ATOVAQUONE/PROGUANIL

Atovaquone/proguanil is a combination of two very old antimalarial drugs, the familiar proguanil (Paludrine) and atovaquone, a distant chemical relative of quinine. The drug is effective both as a malaria prophylactic and cure, and is thought to have less in the way of side effects than many other antimalarials. It is available in North America, Western Europe and a number of developing countries. Although licensed mostly for treatment, it is an effective prophylactic, and has the advantage of needing to be taken for only seven days after leaving a malarious area. Most other prophylactics need to be taken for four weeks after departing the malaria risk area.

IMMUNISATION

Although much work has been done in the development of a vaccine, we are still many years away from the release and active use of a universally applicable vaccine.

Different populations are likely to need different vaccines e.g. residents of malarious areas will require a different vaccine to short-stay tourists.

To date, no truly exciting candidate vaccine against malaria has come along. A number of vaccines have undergone tropical field trials, but it is unlikely that any will remove the need for chemoprophylaxis in the near future.

Recent trials have demonstrated a reduction in severe malaria by around 30 to 40% in children living in high risk areas. Although this is a breakthrough of sorts, it does not address the needs in any way of the visitor to malaria areas.

UNTREATABLE MALARIA

The most frightening prospect of all, untreatable malaria, is continuously mentioned in connection with countries in South-east Asia. Strains of malaria have evolved in this region, particularly along the Thai-Myanmar (Burma) border, that have shown resistance to all conventional drugs. Civil unrest and war have exacerbated the problem.

Despite the existence of so-called untreatable malaria, researchers believe that all malaria can be treated and cured, but this may now require a combination of drugs rather than relying on the administration of only one kind of drug. Indeed, the use of judiciously selected drug combinations has shown some promise in this area.

Diligent management of the resources used to fight malaria, as well as strict control of drug availability, will be required to make headway in the fight against malaria. The WHO-inspired Multilateral Initiative on Malaria and Roll Back Malaria campaigns include better drug management in their aims.

24

HIV/AIDS AND MALARIA

When people who are living with HIV contract other infections, two major problems can arise:

- The infection will be more serious because the person's immune system is not working properly
- The new infection will make the HIV itself worse by increasing the person's viral load – this is a measure of the number of viruses in an infected person's system, and an indicator of current status.

In the case of malaria, both of these factors are a concern.

IS MALARIA MORE SERIOUS IN AN HIV-INFECTED PERSON?
The answer is now clear – Yes.

For some years, we thought that malaria was not really a disease that behaved opportunistically, that took advantage of a person's weakened immune system.

However, many studies have now demonstrated that people with existing HIV infection are at risk of severe malaria – both travellers and people who have previously acquired semi-immunity during childhood in high risk areas.

When the immune system starts to malfunction, the protection conferred upon semi-immune individuals disappears – and instead of being in a position where they have malaria parasites in the blood and are well, they become ill with clinical malaria. As not all the components of the human immune response to malaria are affected by the HIV virus, this weakening of the immune system varies from individual to individual. What has also been noted is that the worse the HIV infection is – as measured by declining CD4 count and increasing viral load – the worse will be the malaria.

Consequently, we can be sure that HIV-infected local residents in a high-risk area will get more severe malaria, more often.

In the case of non-immune persons with HIV visiting high-risk areas, the risk is greater of complicated malaria and death. As there is absolutely no pre-existing immunity, malaria may present in these individuals as a rapidly progressing and overwhelming infection.

A recently discovered phenomenon is that people living with AIDS might have a poorer response to treatment with some malaria drugs – artemesinins and sulphadoxine/pyrimethamine specifically.

In summary – HIV infection makes clinical malaria more likely to occur in local residents, while in visitors it is more likely to cause severe disease and death.

DOES MALARIA MAKE PRE-EXISTING HIV INFECTION WORSE?

The answer here is also yes. We measure the activity of HI Virus in a person's body in a number of ways. One of these is to use a technique that estimates the number of viruses in circulation in an affected person's blood.

During the initial latent or 'quiet' stage of HIV infection, the number of viruses circulating is relatively low. When malaria occurs, the number increases markedly and this may accelerate the progress of the disease.

In those HIV-infected persons who have developed clinical AIDS, a similar phenomenon occurs – worsening the already present diseases.

Increasing viral loads has a number of clinical and public health implications – it may increase the risk of mother-to-child HIV transmission, or impact on resistance patterns to anti-retroviral treatments – to name just a couple.

WHAT ABOUT PEOPLE WHO ARE TAKING ANTI-AIDS DRUGS?

Unfortunately, some of the treatments used for malaria conflict with anti-retroviral (ARV) medication.

Dangerous interactions can occur between the protease inhibitor (PI) group of ARV drugs and commonly used malaria treatments, such as artemether, atovaquone, proguanil, lumefantrine and artesunate. This also occurs with delaviridine, a so-called NNRTI drug.

Other drugs can cause interference with the absorption and metabolism of the antimalarial drug, and prevent the drug from reaching active levels in the blood.

Theoretically, PIs and NNRTIs can also interfere with quinine, the gold standard of malaria treatment.

WHAT DOES THIS MEAN FOR HIV-INFECTED TRAVELLERS?

- Ideally, those living with HIV should not expose themselves to the risk of malaria.
- If the risk exposure is unavoidable, they should speak to their HIV caregiver and travel clinic regarding the best preventative strategy.
- Employers should inform all their workers about the risk of working in malaria areas while living with HIV.
- Disclosure to the attending physician of the person's HIV status is essential to allow for proper planning of treatment, should malaria be contracted.

WHAT DOES THIS MEAN FOR THOSE LIVING IN A MALARIA AREA WHO ARE HIV INFECTED?

- Those people who were previously regarded as being semi-immune, and have subsequently become HIV positive, are at risk of clinical malaria.
- HIV-positive pregnant women and children are especially at risk.

APPENDIX 1: TREATMENT OPTIONS

Not everyone reading this book will have to decide for himself or herself which drug to take for treatment or as a prophylaxis. However, there will be those who need to have such information at hand, merely because other information sources are not readily available or because they wish to expand on information they may already have obtained from their doctor.

WARNING

It is intended that in all cases where medical help is available, the patient should attempt to obtain it and not treat himself. No responsibility will be taken by the author or publisher for any negative consequences arising out of advice taken from this book.

THE MOST IMPORTANT ASPECTS OF TREATMENT

- Prompt and effective treatment with antimalarials.
- Correction of fluid and electrolyte substances if there has been a fluid loss.
- Correction of hypoglycaemia or low blood sugar, especially in diabetics and pregnant women.
- Correction of anaemia.
- Treatment of concurrent infection if one exists.

WHEN TO TREAT FOR MALARIA

If *P. falciparum* is suspected, even if test results are not yet available or are negative, if the patient has fever or any of the common signs of malaria (see pages 38–41), antimalarial treatment must be given. If any other illness is suspected at the same time, treat for that as well.

THE MOST IMPORTANT AIM IN TREATMENT

The most important aim in treatment is to bring the level of parasites present in the blood *under control as quickly as possible* by the administration of rapidly acting drugs. This presents little difficulty except in *P. falciparum* malaria, where the progression of the disease is extremely rapid.

THE DIFFERENT TYPES OF TREATMENT DRUGS AVAILABLE

The name in the column on the left in Table 5 is the generic name, commonly used by doctors and medical personnel. The names in the middle column are likely to be more familiar to the public.

This is an area of potentially major confusion when one drug is given more than one trade name or when patients do not understand to which drug their doctor is referring.

Trade names also differ in different countries. Some treatment drugs are used as prophylactics while others are used exclusively for treatment, and still others are used for both.

Table 5: Malaria drugs and their role in treatment

Drug	Brand name	Comment
Quinine	Quinine	Drug of choice
Quinidine	Quinidine	May be used instead of quinine
Artemether	Artemether	Effective with mefloquine
Artemether-benflumetol	Riamet, Co-Artem	Effective
Artesunate	Artesunate	Effective with mefloquine
Atovaquone-proguanil	Atovaquone/proguanil	Effective
Mefloquine	Lariam, Mefliam, Mephaquin	Effective
Sulphadoxine-pyrimethamine	Fansidar	Widespread resistance

Drug	Brand name	Comment
Doxycycline	Vibramycin, many others	In combination with quinine
Clindamycin	Dalacin	In combination with quinine
Halofantrine	Halfan	Cardiotoxic, unreliable
Primaquine	Primaquine	Elimination of relapsing malaria
Chloroquine	Nivaquine, Avloclor, others	Very limited indications for use
Amodiaquine	Camoquin, Flavoquin, Basoquin	Side effects may occur

QUININE

This is the drug of choice to treat *P. falciparum* malaria. It is the gold standard by which all others are judged. It is best administered together with either tetracycline or clindamycin to prevent the development of resistance.

Because of the serious nature of malaria caused by *P. falciparum* and the reliability of quinine, it is commonly employed as the first line of treatment. Whenever severe *P. falciparum* malaria is encountered, it is preferable that quinine be given intravenously until the infection has been brought under control. Once it has been, and the patient can take medication by mouth, then it is given orally. Quinine is administered either orally or by injection. It is extremely valuable because of its rapid action on parasites.

Some resistance to quinine has developed, particularly in Thailand where it has been used extensively for malaria therapy. Whenever it is used, it should be under medical or hospital supervision.

Contraindications

Quinine should not be used in those with a history of hypersensitivity to quinine, and used with caution in certain types of heart disease and people taking anti-coagulants.

Side effects

Side effects in many patients include giddiness, light-headedness, temporary hearing loss, tinnitus (ringing in the ears) and blurred vision.

Anorexia (loss of appetite), nausea and vomiting may occur after the first few doses although these may be difficult to distinguish from the symptoms of acute malaria.

Less frequent but more serious effects of quinine include abnormal cardiac rhythms, thrombocytopenia (low platelet count), haemolysis (destruction of red blood cells) and oedema (increase in tissue fluids) of the eyelids, mucous membranes and lungs. These may occur following a single dose and necessitate immediate discontinuation of the drug.

Repeat administration of quinine in full therapeutic doses may give rise to a train of symptoms known as 'cinchonism', characterized by tinnitus, headache, nausea, abdominal pain, pruritus, other skin rashes, disturbed vision and even temporary blindness. Some patients are hypersensitive to quinine and even small doses may give rise to symptoms of cinchonism, asthma and other allergic phenomena.

Hypoglycaemia (low blood sugar) due to malaria may be aggravated by oral treatment of even low doses of quinine, as a result of stimulation of insulin secretion. This is a particularly important consideration in the treatment of malaria in pregnant women, whose blood glucose should be carefully monitored.

Quinine treatment was at one time thought to be risky in pregnancy. This is now known not to be the case, however, and it is considered the drug of choice for treating pregnant women with malaria. What were previously thought to be signs of foetal distress associated with the use of quinine are now more properly attributed to the presence of fever and other effects of malaria itself.

QUINIDINE

Quinidine may be used instead of quinine where quinine is unobtainable, as in the USA where it is not registered. It is to all intents and purposes virtually identical to quinine.

TETRACYCLINE AND DOXYCYCLINE

Doxycycline is a long-acting form of tetracycline that many doctors feel offers more convenient dosing than plain tetracycline. These drugs are effective but slow blood schizonticides (meaning that they kill maturing parasites in the bloodstream). Although they can be used alone as prophylaxis against malaria, they should never be used in this way for treatment, and must always be taken in combination.

They are usually administered orally with the more fast-acting quinine so that initial control of parasite levels and symptoms is established. The combination reduces potential quinine toxicity and the emergence of resistance. It has proved useful in areas where quinine resistance is a concern.

Tetracycline and doxycycline are usually given orally and should not be given to pregnant women or to children under the age of eight, except when the risk of withholding the drug outweighs the risk of damage to developing teeth and bones.

Side effects

The most commonly experienced side effects of tetracycline or doxycycline administration are gastrointestinal, including epigastric distress, abdominal discomfort, nausea, vomiting and diarrhoea, as well as photosensitivity, a side effect in which the skin becomes extremely sensitive to sunlight.

Gastrointestinal distress is best avoided by taking tetracycline or doxycycline during daytime. Doxycycline in particular should be washed down with copious fluids, and patients should remain upright if possible after administration.

CLINDAMYCIN

This is an antibiotic used in combination with quinine, when tetracycline or doxycycline is contraindicated, as in pregnancy. It too should not be used alone, and is not used for prophylaxis. Clindamycin may rarely be associated with a severe form of antibiotic-associated diarrhoea.

MEFLOQUINE (LARIAM, MEFLIAM, MEPHAQUIN)

Related chemically to quinine, mefloquine is effective against many parasites that are resistant to other drugs. It can be used as a treatment or for prophylaxis, even on a long-term basis.

The dosage of mefloquine for treatment is 15 mg/kg immediately, followed by another 10 mg/kg eight to 24 hours later.

Side effects

The main adverse reactions are dizziness, disturbed balance, nausea, vomiting, diarrhoea, abdominal pain and loss of appetite.

Effects are mild to moderate and do not require specific treatment. Severe dizziness has been reported in certain individuals.

There are reports of serious adverse neurological and psychiatric effects following both the therapeutic and prophylactic use of mefloquine. These reactions have ranged from fatigue, weakness and malaise, to seizures and acute psychosis.

Caution is advised by some experts in the use of mefloquine in patients concurrently taking beta-blockers and certain calcium channel blockers. There is agreement that mefloquine is best avoided with drugs that affect heart rhythm, such as digitalis. Epileptics should not take mefloquine, and neither should people with any history of mental illness, such as depression.

Those who need fine motor co-ordination in the course of their employment or travel, such as pilots and divers, should avoid this drug for prophylaxis.

Safety data supports the use of mefloquine as prophylaxis in the second and third trimesters of pregnancy, and limited data lends similar support for prophylactic use in the first trimester. When used to treat pregnant women with malaria, the higher doses of mefloquine have been associated with a higher than expected rate of miscarriage.

The drug should not be used in children weighing less than 5 kg, and in people suffering from epilepsy or a psychiatric disorder.

ATOVAQUONE/PROGUANIL

This drug, a combination of two old and well-known antimalarials, is effective as oral treatment for *P. falciparum* malaria and has demonstrated efficacy and safety when used as a prophylactic. It is indicated for the treatment of uncomplicated malaria where resistance to other drugs is a problem. Resistance to this drug is starting to emerge in parts of West Africa.

ARTEMESININS

This group of drugs should never be used alone to treat malaria, as dangerous recrudescences can occur. They have been successfully used in combination with both mefloquine (Lariam, Mefliam, Mephaquin) and benflumetol (lumafantrine).

In those countries where artemesinins are sold alone, and not in combination, it would be wise to combine them with mefloquine (Lariam, Mefliam, Mephaquin).

CO-ARTEMETHER (CO-ARTEM, RIAMET)

A combination of artemether and benflumetol, co-artemether is indicated for the treatment of uncomplicated malaria. The artemether causes rapid improvement in symptoms, knocking out most of the malaria parasites in the bloodstream, while the benflumetol mops up any resistant parasites that evaded elimination by the artemether. Treatment is oral, and is generally well tolerated.

SULPHADOXINE-PYRIMETHAMINE (FANSIDAR)

At one stage, the drug Fansidar (sulphadoxine-pyrimethamine) was in favour as a first-line treatment against *P. falciparum* malaria. This is, however, no longer considered a first-line drug. Toxicity, as well as widespread resistance, have led to its fall from favour. Medical practitioners now prefer to use the more reliable quinine to treat malaria caused by *P. falciparum*.

Side effects

Sulphadoxine-pyrimethamine (Fansidar) is capable of producing severe adverse reactions in some people, especially those who are allergic to sulpha drugs. Severe allergic reactions may cause death.

Others who should not use Fansidar are:

- newborn infants.
- women in the later stages of pregnancy.
- persons with kidney or liver disorders.
- people with a history of allergy to sulpha drugs.
- people with porphyria.

Its use has been linked with bone-marrow suppression, usually with prolonged dosage. The more widespread use of Fansidar as a treatment in recent times has led to an increased resistance to it.

It was previously used as a prophylactic but its use was associated with severe and sometimes fatal skin rashes. When used for treatment, it is administered as a single dose:

under 4 years	½ tablet
4-8 years	1 tablet
9-14 years	2 tablets
over 14 years	3 tablets

(Confirm with a local doctor, if at all possible.)

CHLOROQUINE

Chloroquine is currently indicated only for the treatment of the very uncommon chloroquine-sensitive *P. falciparum,* and against *P. malariae.* It is also used to terminate acute attacks of *P. vivax* or *P. ovale* malaria.

Because chloroquine has antipyretic properties, it acts in the same manner as aspirin to reduce fever. This is why people may feel temporarily better, while the malaria is in fact still multiplying in the system. This makes its use dangerous in chloroquine- resistant areas.

The tablets usually contain 150 mg of chloroquine base per tablet. For a malaria attack, a total course of treatment would comprise 25 mg/kg, usually given orally in a three-day course for the treatment of chloroquine-sensitive *P. falciparum*.

The standard regimen consists of 10 mg base/kg of body weight followed by 5 mg/kg six to eight hours later and 5 mg/kg on each of the second and third days (WHO *Practical Chemotherapy of Malaria*). To eliminate the risk of nausea and vomiting, do not take on an empty stomach.

Table 6 gives the total amount of chloroquine to be taken over three days according to body weight.

Table 6: Chloroquine dosages

5 kg	125 mg	just over ½ tablet
10 kg	250 mg	just over ¾ tablet
15 kg	375 mg	one tablet and ¼
20 kg	500 mg	one tablet and ⅔
30 kg	750 mg	two tablets and ½
40 kg	1 000 mg	three tablets and ⅓
50 kg	1 250 mg	four tablets and under ¼
60 kg	1 500 mg	five tablets
70 kg	1 750 mg	five tablets and over ¾
80 kg	2 000 mg	six tablets and ⅔
90 kg	2 250 mg	seven tablets and ½
100 kg	2 500 mg	eight tablets and ⅓
110 kg	2 750 mg	nine tablets

Chloroquine resistance

Resistance to chloroquine by *P. falciparum* has spread to most areas of the world. Only limited areas in North Africa, the Middle East, Central America, and the Caribbean still boast chloroquine sensitivity. Once a drug starts to fail in 25% of cases treated in a particular region, it is usually abandoned in favour of others.

This is the situation with chloroquine in most areas of the world where *P. falciparum* is a threat.

Contraindications

Chloroquine should not be used:

- if malaria is contracted in an area where chloroquine resistance occurs (most of the world's malarious areas).
- when an infection has broken through despite the use of chloroquine as a prophylactic (use as prophylactic is declining on account of increasing resistance).
- if malaria appears unresponsive to treatment with chloroquine.
- in patients with impaired liver or kidney function, careful dosing is required.
- in patients with retinal disease.
- in patients with porphyria or psoriasis. Alcoholics tend to have an adverse reaction to chloroquine.

Side effects

Adverse effects are rare and mild when the drug is given orally in the usual antimalarial doses. Nausea and vomiting may occur if it is taken on an empty stomach. Headache and visual difficulties have been reported in patients receiving a therapeutic regimen of 25 mg/kg. Pruritus, or itching of palms, soles and scalp has been reported in up to 20% of Africans using chloroquine, a condition that is not relieved by antihistamines. All these side effects are reversible upon discontinuation of the medication.

Symptoms of poisoning by overdosage include headache, nausea, diarrhoea, dizziness, muscular weakness, blurred vision, and a slow pulse. Overdosing with chloroquine is extremely dangerous and requires intensive hospital care if the patient is to be saved.

HALOFANTRINE (HALFAN)

This drug has been associated with unexpected cardiac arrest and sudden death. It is also unpredictably absorbed from the intestine into the bloodstream. Although widely available in the third world, its use outside sophisticated settings where cardiac monitoring is available is to be avoided.

AMODIAQUINE (CAMOQUIN)

Amodioquine is an older drug that has side effect-related problems, but it is seeing something of a resurgence. Used in smaller quantities at lower dosage, it has been accepted as a combination drug to be used with artemesinins.

Side effects

Like chloroquine, Camoquin causes pruritus. It also carries the risks of toxic hepatitis and potentially lethal agranulocytosis (white blood cells stop being produced). It may cause severe suppression of the bone marrow when used for prophylaxis over a long period.

PRIMAQUINE

Primaquine is highly effective against gametocytes and against the latent liver stages of relapsing malarias but has little blood (schizontocidal) activity. This means that it is more useful for treating the relapsing malarias as caused by *P. ovale* and *P. vivax*.

The usual dose for anti-relapse therapy of *P. vivax* and *P. ovale* is 15 mg base daily for 14 days. A dose of chloroquine is usually given first to kill the acute phase of the disease.

Toxic symptoms are rare when primaquine is given at the usual dosage. Primaquine should be given with extreme care to patients being treated with myeloid depressant drugs or who suffer from bone-marrow suppression, from whatever cause.

Contraindications

Patients with a genetic deficiency of the enzyme G-6-P-D should only use primaquine under the supervision of an expert, to avoid serious haematological complications. It is essential to do a blood test to detect any G-6-P-D deficiency before treatment. Primaquine should be avoided in pregnancy in case the foetus is G-6-P-D-deficient.

DRUG RESISTANCE DEFINED

Resistance describes the parasite's ability to withstand the effects of a drug. This reduces the drug's ability to cure the disease. Resistance occurs under the following conditions:

- widespread use of the drug.
- insufficient dosage.
- partial administration of the course of drugs.

When insufficient dosage and partial administration take place, the parasites in the bloodstream are said to be 'selected' for resistance. That means that the stronger parasites, which are able to overcome the limited effect of the drug, survive to breed more of their kind, while the weaker ones that succumb to the drug die out, leaving behind only the resistant parasites.

The parasites will breed and sooner or later a new infection will beak through and require treatment.

The next time the drug is taken, its job will be much harder as it will have to fight against resistant parasites. The chances are that it will fail in its task.

CONDITIONS REQUIRING SPECIAL CARE IN MEDICATION

- *Sulpha-sensitive patients* should definitely avoid Maloprim, Fansidar, and Lap-Dap.
- *Cardiac patients*: quinidine is more likely to cause cardiac rhythm disturbances than quinine. Halofantrine (Halfan) has been associated with cardiac arrest and sudden death. Mefloquine should be used with caution in combination with digitalis, some beta-blockers, and certain calcium-channel blockers.
- *Patients with liver disorders* should use tetracycline and doxycycline under expert guidance.
- *Patients with kidney disorders* should avoid tetracycline, although they may use doxycycline.

- *Pregnant women's* blood glucose must be carefully monitored for hypoglycaemia if quinine is used as treatment; mefloquine may be associated with an increased risk of miscarriage when used for the treatment of malaria. Do not take primaquine, because of potential harm to the foetus. Sulpha-containing drugs such as Fansidar (sulphadoxine-pyrimethamine), Maloprim (dapsone-pyrimethamine), and Lap-Dap (chlorproguanil and dapsone) are best avoided in late pregnancy. Proguanil (Paludrine), chlorproguanil (Lapudrine), pyrimethamine, dapsone, and sulphadoxine should all be supplemented with folic acid if they are used in pregnancy.
- *Epileptics* should not take mefloquine, and should also avoid chloroquine if at all possible.
- *Depressive patients or others with a psychiatric history* should avoid mefloquine. A history of use of any antidepressant, including popular drugs such as Prozac (fluoxetine) precludes the use of mefloquine.
- *Those who have had repeated, frequent malaria attacks,* particularly if there is a suspicion of treatment failure, need specialized care.
- *G-6-P-D deficient patients* should not take primaquine, except under specialized care.
- Porphyria sufferers should not take sulpha-containing drugs such as Fansidar (sulphadoxine-pyrimethamine), Maloprim (dapsone-pyrimethamine) and Lap-Dap (chlorproguanil-dapsone). They should also avoid tetracycline, doxycyline, and chloroquine. Mefloquine is safe in porphyria.

WHY IT IS IMPORTANT TO TAKE THE ENTIRE COURSE OF TREATMENT
If only a proportion of the entire treatment dosage is taken, enough to kill off a sufficient number of parasites to eliminate symptoms of the disease, but not enough to kill all the parasites in the blood, this will result in the recurrence of the malaria in a few weeks' time when the parasites have had a chance to build up to levels that overcome the body's immune system.

Another effect of not taking a sufficient dosage or the full course of treatment is that the parasites are selected that are less sensitive to the drug. If these multiply, a new strain of resistant parasite, which is immune to that drug, becomes more widespread.

THE HIERARCHY OF DRUG DEFENCE
Here one needs to distinguish between a country's drug and prescription policy and the options open to the individual. Official facilities may not always offer the most effective treatment.

In areas where drug resistance is a problem, it may be wise to travel equipped with a supply of an effective drug.

Quinine in combination with another drug, usually doxycycline, remains the treatment of choice in most regions, while Atovaquone/proguanil, mefloquine (Lariam, Mefliam, Mephaquin), and co-artemether (Co-Artem, Riamet) may be useful alternatives.

WHAT IF IT DOESN'T WORK?
It will be seen within 48 hours that symptoms have not been relieved, that the fever is still occurring at intervals and that the patient's condition is deteriorating. It is usual to retest the blood for a parasite count and then change the course of therapy. However, many factors are at play here including the parasite's sensitivity to the drug used.

WHAT IF YOU WAIT TOO LONG TO TREAT MALARIA?
Unless malaria is treated immediately, symptoms will be extreme and the more complicated forms of malaria may arise: certainly there is a high risk of anaemia and cerebral malaria as well as the risk of kidney failure.

The patient must be hospitalized and treatment for the various complications given. There is a highly significant correlation between the delay in starting treatment and death. To have any impact on a patient, chemotherapy must be started as soon as possible.

WHAT ARE THE CONSEQUENCES OF SELF-MEDICATION?

If the correct drug is used – and the appropriate dosage given in good enough time – the chances are that the patient will recover. However, there is always a risk that the patient is given too little or too much of a drug, or that a particular drug is selected to which the parasites are already resistant.

Probably the most common and the most serious consequence of unsuccessful self-medication is delay in seeking treatment. With malaria, a delay of four days can prove fatal.

An average of 2.8 days between the onset of symptoms and death was found in children in The Gambia, although it is not known why some died much sooner.

THE DANGERS OF SELF-MEDICATION

- You might choose the right drug but the incorrect dosage for your body weight.
- The confusing range of drugs that can be taken mean that you might start medication with one type of tablet and switch to another if symptoms do not improve. The new drug may be just a different form of the same drug and therefore be as ineffective as the first drug. In the meantime, the malaria will have progressed and your condition will have deteriorated.
- Overdosage: you might start to take a drug, not feel better, visit a doctor and omit to tell him you have taken the drug. He may give you a drug that, when taken in combination with the drug you have already taken, results in overdosage or incompatibility and consequently serious side effects.
- Self-medication with antimalarials may be used for symptoms that are not malaria at all resulting in a situation where other causes of fever will go undetected and untreated.

Rehydration

Rehydration is vital in hot climates. Patients with fever may become dehydrated very quickly, especially if they are vomiting and have diarrhoea simultaneously.

Children are especially at risk from dehydration. They are likely to be intolerant of fasting and may therefore become hypoglycaemic. Glucose supplements included in oral rehydration formulas for the control of diarrhoea may help control the hypoglycaemia.

Where vomiting or dehydration is not present, it is sufficient for cool liquids to be given. It is important to note that alcoholic beverages worsen dehydration. Where vomiting or diarrhoea is present, give the commercially available, specially formulated oral rehydration therapy (ORT) powder, which is mixed with cooled, boiled water. This formulation contains salts and sugars to replace those that were lost through vomiting and diarrhoea.

If you have no access to specially formulated powders, make up your own. This consists of one teaspoon of salt and six tablespoons of sugar in one litre of cooled, boiled water (see also dehydration remedy on page 48). This is likely to be unpalatable to children who may prefer to take diluted, flat Coca-Cola. Never give milk or other dairy products to a person with vomiting and diarrhoea.

Bed rest and lowering of body temperature may reduce vomiting and allow patients to be treated orally. If the frequency of vomiting and diarrhoea is such that it prevents the patient from keeping down fluids and medicine, such a patient should be hospitalized and administered liquid through a drip.

Reducing fever

Fever needs to be reduced to control the risk of convulsions, especially in young children. Typically, malaria produces high fevers of 39 °C and above.

Physical methods, such as the removal of clothes, fanning and sponging with lukewarm water are the most reliable.

Various anti-fever drugs are used in the treatment of malaria patients. Paracetamol is preferred to aspirin and it can be given by mouth or suppository. Suppositories are indicated for infants or children, or where vomiting is preventing the absorption of the drug. Crushed tablets can be administered via nasogastric tube.

Combating anaemia

As more and more red blood cells are destroyed by the malaria parasites, the blood's oxygen-carrying capacity decreases.

Chronic and progressive anaemia are major problems associated with malaria, particularly in children and pregnant women. In cases where the oxygen content of the blood is reduced beyond a critical point, blood transfusions may be needed. Of course, this presents major problems in areas where blood is not routinely screened for HIV, or is not available.

Tourists and travellers to malaria-endemic areas are advised to know their blood group, and if possible to draw up a list of potential blood donors with whom they are familiar, and whom they can trust not to have AIDS. A number of organisations, including the Blood Foundation in the United Kingdom, now undertake to rush safe blood to most developing countries when needed. Arrangements with these organisations usually need to be made in one's home country before departure.

Table 7: Information required by doctor before treatment

- Which species of malaria parasite is prevalent in country of destination?
  [ ] *falciparum*   [ ] *vivax*   [ ] *malariae*   [ ] *ovale*

- Which drug was used for chemoprophylaxis during visit?

- When did you first start taking the chemoprophylaxis?
  Date: . . . .

- When did you stop taking the chemoprophylaxis?
  Date: . . . .

- How often was it taken?
  [ ] once a week   [ ] daily   [ ] other . . . .

- Did you take it conscientiously and at about the same time every day
  or week?

- At what dosage was it taken?
  [ ] one tablet   [ ] two tablets   [ ] other . . . .

- Is there any aspect of your medical history that should be noted by a
  doctor prescribing drugs for the treatment of malaria?
  [ ] pregnancy   [ ] hypoglycaemia   [ ] hepatitis
  [ ] kidney disorder   [ ] sulpha sensitivity   [ ] porphyria
  [ ] cardiac condition   [ ] depressive condition
  [ ] other . . . .

- What other medicines are you taking?

Table 8: Information necessary for prescribing antimalarials to travellers

- Which species of malaria parasite is prevalent in country of destination?
  [ ] *falciparum* [ ] *vivax* [ ] *malariae* [ ] *ovale*

- Drug sensitivity list: Which drugs work best for treatment in country of destination?

- Is there any aspect of your medical history that should be noted by a doctor prescribing drugs for the prevention of malaria?
  [ ] pregnancy   [ ] hypoglycaemia   [ ] hepatitis
  [ ] kidney disorder   [ ] sulpha sensitivity   [ ] porphyria
  [ ] cardiac condition [ ] depressive condition
  [ ] other . . . .

- What other medicines are you taking?

APPENDIX 2: PROPHYLAXIS

WARNING

Remember that no drug is 100% effective. Even though you may comply with the drug dosage instructions, you may still contract malaria. Drug prophylaxis remains controversial and recommendations change constantly.

CHEMOPROPHYLAXIS AND STAND-BY MEDICATION

The following summarizes the situation when chemoprophylaxis and stand-by treatment may be considered; detailed recommendations are given in *International Travel and Health Vaccination Requirements and Health Advice* (published by the WHO).

Chemoprophylaxis and stand-by medicament are not recommended in areas where transmission of malaria has not been reported or occurs only at a very low level, and where suitable diagnostic and therapeutic facilities are within easy reach.

Chemoprophylaxis is not recommended but stand-by medicament is to be available in areas where transmission of malaria is low and diagnosis and therapeutic facilities are not readily available.

Chemoprophylaxis is recommended but stand-by medicament is not required in areas where chemoprophylaxis would be expected to be successful. These are areas with chloroquine-sensitive *P. falciparum* and areas with *P. vivax* or *P. malariae* or both but without *P. falciparum*. Chloroquine is the prophylactic of choice but an alternative drug needs to be carried.

Both chemoprophylaxis and stand-by medicament are recommended for travellers to areas where a reasonable risk of infection with *P. falciparum* exists, and where the drug used for prophylaxis may not be effective in preventing clinical illness.

The consensus of opinion among malaria experts is that where a risk of infection with *P. falciparum* exists, chemoprophylaxis and personal protection measures must both be employed to protect against malaria.

Table 9: Drugs for prophylaxis

Drug	Brand name	Comment
Mefloquine	Lariam, Mefliam, Mephaquin	Effective, but observe contraindications
Doxycycline	Vibramycin, many others	Effective, but observe contraindications
Atovaquone-proguanil	Atovaquone/proguanil	Effective
Chloroquine	Aralen, Avloclor, Nivaquine, Delagil, Lagaquin, Larigo, Malaviron, Resochin, Starquine	Widespread resistance by *P. falciparum*. Even in combination with proguanil is considered less effective in most areas
Proguanil	Paludrine	Used in combination with chloroquine, but not highly effective. Not available in USA
Chloroquine-proguanil	Daramal and Paludrine	Not highly effective
Chloroquine-pyrimethamine	Daraclor	Not highly effective
Dapsone-pyrimethamine	Maloprim	Not highly effective, problems with toxicity

MEFLOQUINE (LARIAM, MEFLIAM, MEPHAQUIN)

An extremely effective prophylactic, this drug is well tolerated by most people, provided the contraindications are observed. It should not be used by anybody with a history of epilepsy, depression, or other psychiatric disorder. It must be used with caution in combination with some cardiac drugs, such as beta-blockers, and is contraindicated in combination with others, such as digitalis and certain calcium-channel blockers. It may also render inactive some of the newer oral vaccines used to protect against typhoid and cholera. The commonest reported side effect is vivid dreams.

The drug is probably the prophylactic of choice in pregnant women. It may be used in children weighing 5 kg or more. Media reports of severe side effects with this drug are thought to reflect poor adherence by prescribers to contraindications rather than inherent drug toxicity. Provided the contraindications are observed, this drug is usually well tolerated.

DOXYCYCLINE

A useful alternative when mefloquine is contraindicated, doxycycline has been used by many travellers for protracted periods without problems. It is contraindicated in pregnant and breastfeeding women, and for prophylaxis in children under the age of 12 years. Common side effects include gastrointestinal disturbances e.g. nausea and diarrhoea, sensitivity to light characterized by exaggerated sunburn, a number of dermatological reactions and vaginal thrush.

ATOVAQUONE/PROGUANIL

This drug is known to be safe and effective as a prophylactic. It is more expensive than other choices, but has the advantage of only needing to be taken for one week after leaving a malarious area, unlike most other antimalarials that need to be taken for four weeks after leaving the risk area. Atovaquone/proguanil will probably find a niche with the frequent short-stay traveller.

CHLOROQUINE

Widespread resistance by *P. falciparum* means that this drug has very limited application as a prophylactic. Certain restricted areas in Central America, the Caribbean, and North Africa are the only areas where chloroquine resistance is not a problem.

PROGUANIL (PALUDRINE)

Formerly taken on its own, proguanil has been safely taken for 40 years. It is now used mainly in combination with other drugs, and is rarely used alone. Proguanil can safely be used during pregnancy and for children and rarely causes side effects. Those frequently reported are mouth ulcers, hair loss, vomiting and abdominal discomfort.

Pregnant women taking proguanil should take a folic acid supplement.

CHLOROQUINE-PROGUANIL

This combination was developed in an effort to extend the useful life of chloroquine. It is not considered highly effective, but is still widely available. In addition, its combination of daily and weekly dosing can be confusing and lead to side effects and inadequate protection. It is gradually falling out of favour.

CHLOROQUINE-PYRIMETHAMINE

Still available in some countries, low efficacy prevents its recommendation as a prophylactic.

DAPSONE-PYRIMETHAMINE

This combination, on sale in many countries, suffers from the twin problems of low efficacy and significant toxicity. Its use as a prophylactic is no longer recommended.

PYRIMETHAMINE

This drug is no longer sufficiently effective to be recommended itself as a prophylactic; despite this, it too is available in many developing countries. The United States Food and Drug Administration believes pyrimethamine may be carcinogenic.

ORIGINAL BIBLIOGRAPHY

Eddleston M., Pierini S.; *Oxford Handbook of Tropical Medicine* (Oxford University Press), New York, 1999.

Katzung B. G.; *Basic and Clinical Pharmacology*, 8th Edition (McGraw-Hill), New York, 2001.

Gilles H. M.; *Management of Severe and Complicated Malaria* (WHO), Geneva, 1991.

International Travel and Health Vaccination Requirements and Health Advice (WHO), Geneva, 2000.

Global Strategy for Malaria Control, A (WHO), Geneva, 1993.

Malaria Diagnosis – New Perspectives (WHO), Geneva, 2000.

Cook G.; *Manson's Tropical Diseases*, 20th Edition (W. B. McSaunders), 1996.

NEW EDITION BIBLIOGRAPHY & FURTHER READING

Cook G., Zumla A., *Manson's Tropical Diseases*, 21st Edition (W.B. Saunders Company), London, 2002.

Eddleston M., Davidson R., et al; *Oxford Handbook of Tropical Medicine*, Second edition (Oxford University Press), New York, 2005

Katzung B.G.; *Basic and Clinical Pharmacology*, 9th edition (Appleton and Lange), New York, 2004

World Health Organisation; *Management of Severe Malaria – a practical handbook*, Second edition (WHO), Geneva, 2000

World Health Organisation; *International Travel and Health 2005* (WHO), Geneva, 2005

INDEX

A

amodiaquine (Camoquin) 121

anaemia 40, 41, 67, 72, 127

    combatting 127

    in pregnancy 72

Anopheles mosquito 15, 31, 32, 34

artemesinins 105, 117

    and AIDS 109

artemether 47

atovaquone 42, 55, 106, 117, 132

B

benflumetol 105

benign malaria 34, 35 *see also*
  Plasmodium vivax

bites

    cause of itch 33

    reduce chance of, 31

blackwater fever 66

blood

    G-6-P-D level 88, 96, 121, 123

    glucose monitoring 73, 123

    low blood sugar *see*
      hypoglycaemia

C

cardiac arest 120

cardiac patients 120, 122

causal prophylactics 42

    atovaquone 42

    primaquine 42

    proguanil 42

cerebral malaria 50, 66, 84–86

    diagnosis 84

    in children 80

    prognosis 86

    symptoms 85

    treatment 85

chemoprophylaxis *see also*
  prophylaxis, treatment, drugs

    and infertility 76

children

    administering drugs 82

    advice to parents 78

    and chloroquine 78, 81

    and malaria 56

    at risk 77–83

    cerebral malaria 80

    complications in treatment 82

    diagnosis 56, 80

as treatment in pregnancy 75

prophylactics *see* prophylaxis

prophylaxis 16, 51, 52, 77, 97, 98,
130–133

    inadequate 58

protection, mechanical 16, 100–101

protective measures 97-99

pulmonary oedema *see* respiratory
distress syndrome, acute

pyrimethamine 47, 81

    and AIDS 109

    as prophylaxis 133

    treatment in pregnancy 75

recrudescence 87 *see also* relapse

recurring malaria 87–88

rehydration 48, 126

relapse 87, 88 *see also* recrudescence

    prevention of 96

resistance

    definition 122

    to antimalarial drugs 22–29

    to chloroquine 68, 118

respiratory distress syndrome,
acute 66

Roll Back Malaria Initiative 104, 107

Q

quartan *see Plasmodium malariae*

questions commonly asked about
malaria 102–03

quinidine 114

quinine 46, 55, 74, 75, 106, 113

    contraindications 113

    side effects 114

    treatment in pregnancy 74

R

rapid diagnostic tests 57

S

schizonts 43

self-treatment 46

    consequences of 125

    dangers of 125

shock 68

simultaneous treatment 126

spleen, enlargement of 65

sporozoites 43

sulphadoxine 47

    and AIDS 109

sulphadoxine-pyrimethamine
(Fansidar) 76, 117

    treatment in pregnancy 76

NOTES

NOTES

NOTES